# Essential Cleansing for Perfect Health

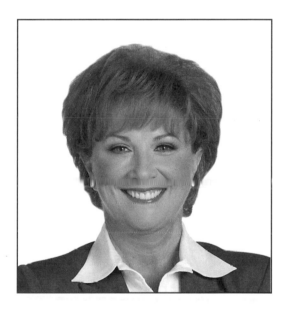

## By Brenda Watson, N.D.

with Suzin Stockton, M.A.

# Essential Cleansing
# for Perfect Health

By Brenda Watson, N.D.

with Suzin Stockton, M.A.

ISBN 0-9719309-1-0

This book is for educational purposes. It is not intended as a substitute for medical advice. Please consult a qualified health care professional for individual health and medical advice. Neither Renew Life Press nor the author shall have any responsibility for any adverse effects arising directly or indirectly as a result of the information provided in this book.

Throughout this book, trademarked names are used. Rather than putting a trademark symbol after every occurrence of a trademarked name, we use names in an editorial fashion only, and to the benefit of the trademark owner, with no intention of infringement of the trademark. Where such designations appear in this book, they have been printed with initial caps.

First Printing
Renew Life Press and Information Services
2076 Sunnydale Drive
Clearwater, FL 33765
1-866-450-1784

# Acknowledgements

There are so many special people that I would like to extend my gratitude and thanks. Due to space constraints within this book, I will only highlight a few from the lengthy list. To the thousands of clients whom I met in clinics and lectures across the country—you are my inspiration for this book.

To all of the people that worked on this book for your hard work—thank you. Suzin Stockton for your help and guidance in creating this book. Your vast knowledge of natural healing and writing contributed greatly to keeping this book on schedule. Steven Beckman for your thoughts and feedback. Paul Pavlovich, for a lovely cover design. To Kathi Murray, Brenda Bellafiore-Valen, and Jerry Adams, without whom this book would not be finished, a special thank you.

To the family of Renew Life and Advanced Naturals, your love and constant support of me and the endeavors of the company make me very grateful and proud. I could not ask for a better support group.

A special thank you to my family and friends who have been instrumental in the process of creating a support system. The most important thank you to my husband, Stan Watson, for his constant support and participation. His endless support has been the reason that I have been able to travel endlessly with this message to thousands of you.

*Brenda Watson*

Brenda Watson, N.D.
Clearwater, FL
2006

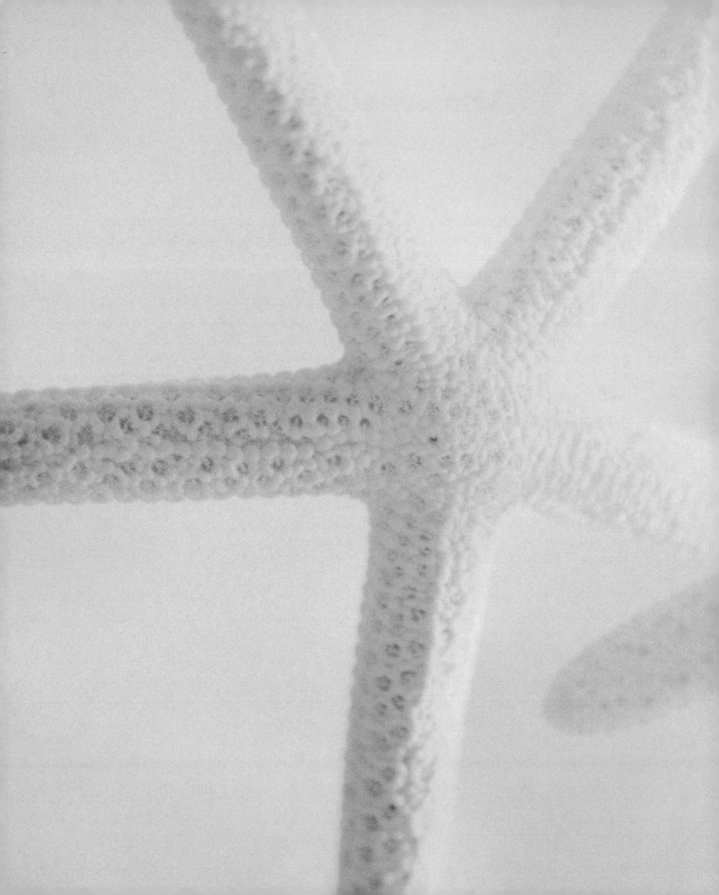

# Preface

After many years of lecturing across the country to thousands of people about the effects of toxicity and the detoxification process, I began to think about writing this book. At each lecture I knew the explanation of the detoxification process needed to be simplified and made "real" to people through the use of pictures and charts. Such visual aids make the information easier to understand.

My personal struggle with poor health made me aware that detoxification is important, whether you're trying to regain health (as I was) or maintain it. In either case, detoxifying the body (ridding it of poisons) and improving the digestive process are necessary.

I regained my health many years ago largely through colon hydrotherapy and herbal supplementation. At that time, such therapeutic practices as fasting and colonics were considered "strange" by most people. The natural healing philosophy has become more accepted during the last two decades, and so too have such therapies. The holistic approach to healing is being increasingly viewed as "scientific" with the accreditation of a growing number of naturopathic colleges.

During my career, I have worked in, and developed, my own clinics that specialize in detoxification and digestive health. In doing so, I have seen many people regain their health and better maintain it through the application of natural healing principles. This has inspired me and given rise to a passion for my work – a passion that remains to this day, which has resulted in a renewed commitment to health education.

I am confident that the information contained in this book will enable you, the reader, to better understand toxicity and the detoxification process. Knowledge is power. The information in Essential Cleansing for Perfect Health will empower you to make the best health choices and quite literally renew your life!

**Brenda Watson, N.D.**

# Table of Contents

# Introduction to
# Toxicity

## The universal symbol for toxicity is the skull and crossbones.

Toxicity, according to the *Cambridge Dictionary of American English*, is "the quality of being poisonous, or the degree to which something is poisonous."[1] A toxin is "a poisonous substance, especially one that is produced by bacteria and causes disease."[2] The dictionary definition of a poison is "a substance that causes illness or death if swallowed, absorbed, or breathed into the body."[3] The words "toxin" and "poison" may therefore be used interchangeably and encompass anything harmful that is taken into or produced in the body, such as bacterial toxins (toxic substances produced by microorganisms), heavy metals, a wide variety of chemicals and more. Interestingly, the word "toxin" has its roots in the Greek word "toxikon," which means poison.[4]

The universal symbol for toxicity is the skull and crossbones. Not all toxic substances are labeled in this manner, however — or labeled at all. While a container of a highly toxic substance, such as lead or arsenic, will likely bear the skull and crossbones symbol, another substance, such as drinking water, which contains trace amounts of these toxins, will not be so marked. While the can of bug spray under your counter will carry a warning on the label, the asparagus you bought from your local supermarket will bear no such warning, despite the fact that it may contain trace amounts of the same (or related) toxic compounds found in the bug spray (a result of pesticide application to commercially grown crops). The dose, of course, makes all the difference. Too often, the difference between the amount of poison that needs a label and a little bit of poison does not compare to the difference between "health" and "illness" for your body, but rather to the difference between "acute" and "chronic" illness.

"Acute" illness is defined as that which has lasted for less than 120 days, as the average cell lives that long".[5] Such illness typically has a sudden onset, sometimes marked by severe symptoms. A cold would be an example of an acute illness. Symptoms that last beyond 120 days are a sign that the illness is being passed from cell to cell and other body systems have become involved. Such chronic illness is characterized by long duration or frequent recurrences (acute flare-ups of chronic conditions). Onset of chronic conditions may be gradual, barely perceivable, in contrast to the explosive onset of acute illness. Conditions such as arthritis and cancer would be examples of chronic illnesses.

Obviously, the higher the exposure to poison, the more symptoms of illness the body will manifest and the more immediate — or acute — will be the response. But, what happens when the dose we take in is so small as to cause no immediate discomfort? Does this mean there is no harm done? Not necessarily. Many toxins accumulate in body tissues. These chemicals are slowly deposited in our bodies, and over time can make us chronically sick if they're allowed to remain there. For this reason, natural health care professionals place a heavy emphasis on toxicity in the body as a major cause of disease.

This perspective stands in contrast to the traditional view held by medicine (the "medical model"), which emphasizes the role of germs as the major factor in many diseases. While the natural healing perspective does not deny the existence of germs, nor the fact that they are often found in patients with disease conditions, it views the presence of these germs more as the result, rather than the cause, of disease. A simple comparison will illustrate this point: Think about a dirty pond filled with mosquitoes. When you see this scene, do you conclude that the mosquitoes caused the pond to be dirty? No, of course not. You know that it was the dirty conditions in the pond that drew the mosquitoes to it. Think of your body as the pond and the mosquitoes as the germs. The message here is that if your body is dirty (internally), it will provide conditions that will attract germs, inviting them to set up housekeeping, and ultimately leading to chronic disease. On the other hand, if your internal environment is clean (relatively free of toxins), germs will likely either have no affect upon you or may only cause short-term discomfort, as conditions are not ripe for them to settle in and multiply.

## Types of Toxins

Broadly speaking, toxins may be divided into two categories, inner and outer. Inner toxins are generated within the body, as opposed to toxins originating outside of the body. Some inner toxin production is the result of normal metabolic processes, meaning that it results from the body's everyday task of converting food to energy.

*While the can of bug spray under your counter will carry a* **warning on the label,** *the vegetables you bought from your local supermarket will bear no such warning.*

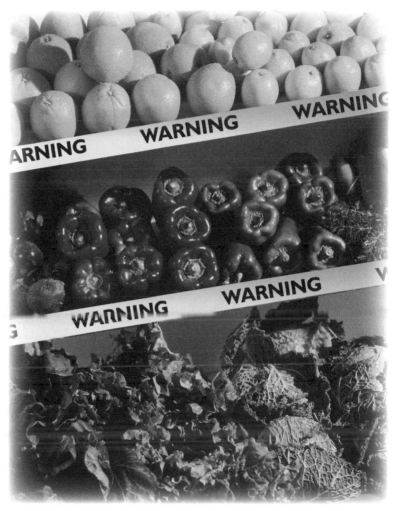

Inner toxins may also be generated as the result of a focal infection anywhere in the body. A focus is a walled-off area of concentrated toxins and dead or infected tissue. The mouth, the begining of the gastrointestinal tract, is commonly a site of such chronic, often silent (producing no local symptoms) infection. The other end of the gastrointestinal tract, the colon, is also a frequent site of inner toxin production.

An outer toxin is simply any toxin generated outside of the human body, one that enters it from the environment, both indoor and outdoor.

# Chapter 1: Environmental Toxins

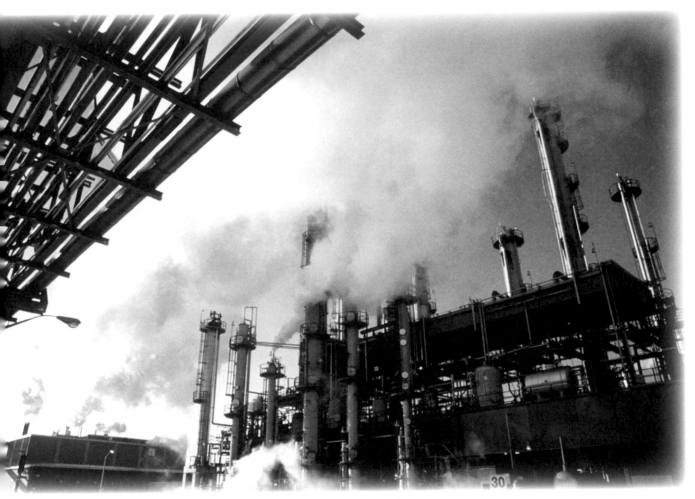

**In 1999, over 20,000 hazardous waste generators, such as chemical manufacturers, photo processing centers, exterminators, dry cleaners, auto repair shops and hospitals, produced over 40 million tons of hazardous waste."**

*Environmental Protection Agency*

Growing environmental toxicity is a topic of world-wide concern today, as the consequences can be catastrophic for the entire planet and its inhabitants. Those consequences express themselves, at least in part, through alarming health statistics.

- **Childhood asthma has increased by more than 40% since 1980.**[1]

- **Fifteen years ago, a half million Americans had Alzheimer's disease. Today five million Americans have it,[2] a number totally out of proportion to the population increase.**

- **In the last decade, the arrest rate of juveniles for murder has increased by 93%.**[3]

- **Cancer is the #2 killer of adults and the #1 cause of death in children. At the beginning of the twentieth century, the incidence of cancer was about 1 in 50. Today, 1 in 3 will suffer from the disease.**[4]

While there is a known genetic component to cancer that is getting a lot of press lately, a recent article posted on the National Cancer Institute's website acknowledges that environmental toxins and lifestyle account for 80-90% of all cancers.[5] Here lifestyle factors would include diet, as well as exposure to infectious agents and pollutants in the air, water and soil. The NCI emphasizes the link between cancer and the environment in *Cancer and the Environment*, a new booklet published jointly with the National Institute of Environmental Health Sciences. Here we have mainstream acknowledgement of what natural healing advocates have stated for years: toxins cause disease!

The pervasiveness of environmental pollution is reflected in the fact that traces of DDT, a chlorine-based pesticide that was banned in the U.S. decades ago, and other chemicals (like PCBs and dioxin) can be found in remote areas of the earth, including the ice at the North Pole. As detoxification expert Sherry Rogers, MD, puts it, "There are no pristine areas left without a trace of man's manufacturing might."[6] DDT was banned because it was found to cause cancer and to persist in the environment. While it's no longer used in the U.S., it is still produced here and exported to other countries, many of which import the DDT-treated food back to us![7]

The measurement of industrial pollutants in air, water and soil by scientists has gone on for decades. Relatively new, however, is a "biomonitoring" process designed to measure the "body burden," or toxic load found in tissues of the human body. This process involves analysis of blood, urine and mother's milk. Using this method, the "first publicly available, comprehensive look at the chemical burden we carry in our bodies" was published in the journal *Public Health Reports* (Thornton, et. al, 2002).[8] The article reported on a classic study led by Mount Sinai School of Medicine in collaboration with the Environmental Working Group and Commonweal that identified 167 chemicals in the blood and urine of nine volunteers who did not work in or live near factories. The bodies of these volunteers stored an average of 91 compounds each (most of which did not exist 75 years ago). Of the 167 chemicals found, 76 are known to cause cancer in humans, 94 are toxic to the brain and nervous system, and 79 cause birth defects or abnormal development.

Many of the damaging pollutants to which we're routinely exposed have been shown to pass through the placenta during pregnancy, thereby gaining entry to the bloodstream of the fetus. A telling study published in the journal *Neurotoxicology* in 2002 found that the first bowel movements of 426 infants from the Philippines showed significant levels of eight different insecticides (including DDT, diazinon, lindane, malathion and

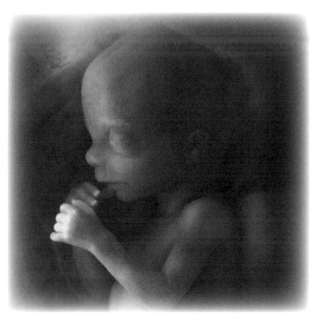

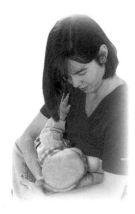

chlordane) and three heavy metals (lead, cadmium and mercury).[9] This study proved that toxic accumulation actually begins before birth. Doris J. Rapp, MD, states the problem as "Unborn babies float nine months in chemicals (DDT and PCBs) in the uterus. Their bowel movements and mother's milk contain the same dangerous pesticides."[10]

PCB stands for polychlorinated biphenyl. Production of these chemicals, used in the manufacture of electronic devices, was banned in 1977, but they persist in the environment and in our bodies. In the period between 1929 and 1977, the U.S. produced over one billion pounds of PCBs; it is estimated that half that amount ended up contaminating the environment.[11] Approximately 312 million pounds are still in use.[12] PCBs are still found extensively in building materials, and large amounts were released on 9/11/01 as a result of the attack on the World Trade Center in New York City.

PCBs, along with heavy metals, pesticides and chemical additives such as bisphenol A (a common plasticizer, a chemical used to make plastics softer, used in the lining of food cans), are *endocrine disrupters*. Endocrine disruptors mimic the body's hormones (especially estrogen), whose job it is to send chemical signals to many organs. Hormone-disrupting chemicals, even at extremely low levels, can have a profoundly damaging effect upon sexual organs and sexual development, including enlarged prostate glands and lower testicular sperm production in males, and early onset of puberty in females.[13] Dr. Rapp reports that PCBs can masculinize females, and that "boys become feminized (undescended testicles, deformed penises and changes in sexuality) from PCBs and dioxin (a chlorine by-product and major component of 'Agent Orange,' the defoliating chemical used extensively in the Vietnam war)".[14] We see this effect in the animal kingdom too, where "low concentrations of these pollutants [endocrine disruptors] are changing both the social and mating behaviors of a raft of species … increasing numbers of male western gulls hatched from eggs exposed to DDT attempt to mate with each other

… while atrazine [a widely used weed killer] makes goldfish hyperactive, and the chemical TCDD [dioxin] makes the play behavior in macaques (a monkey found in Asia and Africa) rougher."[15]

## Environmental toxins can be broadly broken down into four categories:

1. Industrial
2. Agricultural
3. Household
4. Medical/Dental

In reality, there is a tremendous amount of overlap in these categories: the consumer products used in the third and fourth categories are manufactured in an industrial setting, as are most of the products used in the second category, agriculture.

# Industrial Toxins

When we think of pollution, visions of factories belching out toxic gases from their smokestacks are likely to come to mind. The industrial age has proven to be a mixed blessing. On the one hand, it has brought technology, innovation and convenience, and on the other, it has liberated unprecedented amounts of toxins into our air, water and soil. A great deal of environmental damage was done before a need for pollution control devices was recognized and acted upon. Even then, pollution was only reduced, not eliminated.

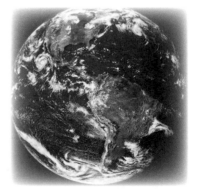

Today's concerns with regard to global warming, as a result of the "Greenhouse Effect" (the rise in temperature that the earth experiences be-cause certain gases in the at-mosphere trap energy from the sun), highlight the negative planetary effects of large-scale industrial production. These concerns become magnified with every report of oil spills, disappearance of rain forests, species extinctions, etc.

The EPA reports that in 2002, 24,379 U.S. facilities released 4.79 billion pounds of toxins into the atmosphere. Of these pollutants, 72 million pounds were known carcinogens.

## Chemicals

Industry has given us thousands of chemicals. Estimates vary between 75,000 and 100,000 now in use, with an additional 1,000 introduced each year. The health effects of very few of these (less than 10%) have been tested. Much could be written (and has been) on these many chemicals, but the focus here will be on pesticides.

These neurotoxins (poisons to the nervous system) are some of the most damaging chemicals in use today due to their pervasiveness and potency. According to Dr. Rapp, "Over 20 studies show pesticides, used inside and outside homes or schools, on lawns or playgrounds, can cause leukemia, brain tumors and lymphomas."[16] The EPA estimates that 74 pesticides, including a number known to cause cancer, presently contaminate the ground water in 38 states.[17] Pesticide products are so extensively used in homes, on farms and by cities in insect abatement programs that these toxins have permeated the environment — and invaded our bodies

*"We were not meant to live on a diet of PCBs, dioxins, pesticides and plastics, yet there are no humans or animals without them."*

*Dr. Sherry A. Rogers, MD, Detoxity or Die, p. 162*

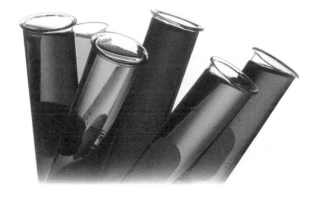

on a grand scale. "A comprehensive survey of more than 1,300 Americans has found traces of weed- and bug-killers in the bodies of everyone tested."[18] Thirteen different pesticides have been found in the body of the average American[19], the same number found in baby foods to which nine out of ten children under age five are exposed.[20] Interestingly, pesticide levels are highest in children and women of childbearing years.[21]

Health effects of the various chemical components of pesticides can be devastating. It has been reported that PCBs may be a contributing cause of Parkinson's disease.[22] Dioxins have been linked to both insulin resistance[23] (inability of the cells to properly use insulin) and diabetes.[24] Other environment-induced diseases that may be linked to pesticides include:[25]

- Cancer, especially breast cancer
- Alzheimer's disease
- Idiopathic peripheral neuropathy (damage to peripheral nerves, unknown origin)
- Neuropsychiatric illnesses (depression, anxiety, forgetfulness, inattention, hyperactivity)
- Chronic fatigue syndrome
- Autoimmune disease, especially lupus
- Allergies, especially eczema

Due to the many contaminants in pesticides, they have the effect of making people more vulnerable to secondary disease and opportunistic infections.

Many of the pesticides discussed fall into the "organophosphate" or "organochloride" categories listed in chart 1, which summarizes "some of the major and most problematic types of hazardous chemicals" in use today, from the perspective of Dr. Doris Rapp, a board-certified specialist in environmental medicine, pediatrics and allergy.

Due to the extensive and long-standing use of potent pesticides and other toxic chemicals, a growing number of people today, including an estimated 74 million Americans,[26] are becoming chemically sensitive. With chemical sensitivity, an exaggerated response to chemicals is displayed. A substantial number (some 10 million) have become so sensitized to chemicals that they can no longer live normally and must take extreme measures to avoid chemical exposure.

# Major Types of Hazardous Chemicals
## Their Sources and Effects

## Organophosphates
(used mostly as insecticides)
Examples: chlorphyrifos, diazinon, parathion, malathion

- Originally designed as nerve gas, damages the nervous system
- May damage lungs, intestines, bladder, heart, muscles, nerves, brain and adversely affect behavior

## Organochlorides - aka chlorinated phenols
(Used mostly as pesticides)
Examples: aldrin, dieldrine, lindane, endrin, atrazine, dioxins, DDT, PBBs (brominated biphenols), the herbicides 2,4-D and 2,4,5-T and the following:

- PCBs can cause cancer, damage the liver, skin and blood, injure the immune, reproductive and nervous systems
- Chloroform, originally used as an anesthetic, is linked to bowel and bladder cancer
- Carbon tetrachloride, trichloroethylene and perchloroethylene are cleaning products that have been known to cause confusion, sleepiness, anesthesia and even death
- Vinyl chloride and ethylene chloride, found in synthetic plastics and cosmetic sprays, can cause liver, brain, intestinal and kidney damage, as well as cancer

## Carbamates
(a category of fungicides and herbicides)
Examples: bendiocarb, carbaryl and aldicarb

- Used in clothing, medicines and plastics
- Can harm lungs, intestines, eyes, brain, muscles, immune and nervous systems
- Can cause: thyroid disturbances, blurred vision, twitches, convulsions, weakness, excessive

perspiration, memory loss, behavior problems, cancer, defective sperm, damage to the unborn.

## Phthalates
(used to soften plastics and extend the life of fragrances)

Sources: industrial chemicals, inks, adhesives, vinyl floor tiles, paints, and plastics

(Phthalates are also found in many beauty care products, including hair spray, shampoo, deodorant, nail polish and perfume; toys; wall coverings; detergents; lubricating oils; plastic wrap; plastic food containers; pharmaceuticals; blood bags and tubing)

- Can cause male offspring of rats to become more feminine and female offspring to have miscarriages
- Can cause early onset of puberty

## Solvents
(used to dissolve the major ingredient in products)
Examples: benzene, toluene and xylene

- Benzene (used in engine fuels and plastic, paint and textile industries) can damage bone marrow and cause leukemia and tumors
- Toluene, used to dissolve many common products, especially printer's ink, damages the nervous system, liver, kidneys, lungs, skin and eyes and can cause developmental delay in children
- Xylene, used in insecticides, plastics, spray paints and inks, as well as in photography, leather and rubber industries, can damage brain, kidneys, eyes, skin and cause numbness of extremities, as well as poor coordination, nauseas and dizziness

Chart 1

From Our Toxic World: A Wake Up Call by Doris J. Rapp, MD, pgs. 13-20

## Heavy Metals

A heavy metal is any metallic element that has a relatively high density — at least five times that of water. Some of the 23 known heavy metals like selenium, copper, manganese and zinc, are nutritional minerals that are needed in small quantities to maintain health but can be toxic at higher doses. Other heavy metals, like arsenic, cadmium, nickel, lead and mercury, are toxic even in small amounts and represent a significant health threat when inhaled, absorbed or ingested, for these elements cannot be degraded or destroyed. Aluminum is another metal that can be toxic to the body, though it doesn't technically meet the definition of heavy metal.

Once toxic metals have accumulated in the body, they're not easily released from storage and flushed from the body. Their continued presence in the tissues of the body creates an ongoing toxic condition that contributes to nutrient deficiency and can lead to serious illness.

Toxic metals tend to accumulate in the immune system and in the brain and kidneys where they can disrupt normal functioning.[28] Once incorporated into tissue, they are difficult to remove because of their density. If not removed, they can be very damaging to the body, as described above.

Before the Industrial age, heavy metals stayed pretty much confined to the interior of the earth, except on rare occasion, such as during a volcanic eruption, when the forces of nature dislodged them. Heavy metals are extensively used today as components of numerous consumer products, though the consumer is generally unaware of their presence in the seemingly harmless product. Since the Industrial Revolution, heavy metal production and distribution have rapidly accelerated, so that the air, water and topsoil of the planet have become permeated with them. These metals tend to persist and accumulate in the environment (and in our bodies!), for they cannot be degraded or destroyed.

We encounter toxic metals every day, as they're widely used in industry, agriculture and food processing. They're even found in some personal care products. Some of the most damaging of the toxic metals are mercury, nickel, lead, cadmium, copper, aluminum, arsenic and platinum. Common sources of these metals are:

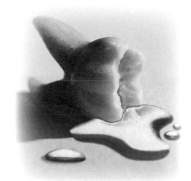

**Mercury:** dental restorations (especially amalgam "silver" fillings), some vaccines (as the preservative thimerosol), thermometers, old paint, pesticides, fish, fluorescent lights, cosmetics, felt, fabric softener and some medicines.

## Drs. Kellas and Dworkin list eight ways in which toxic metals can damage our bodies:[27]

**1.** They can interfere with mineral balance by taking the place of nutritive minerals.

**2.** They disrupt normal metabolic processes.

**3.** Some metal salts, like mercury, have an antibiotic effect, and, like pharmaceutical antibiotics, can destroy beneficial, as well as harmful bacteria, leading to lowered immunity.

**4.** Metals can bind to the body's protein and may trigger an allergic (autoimmune) response when the body fails to recognize its own protein.

**5.** They can initiate free radical damage to cells.

**6.** They can block detoxification pathways.

**7.** Some metals, especially nickel, adversely affect the genetic material RNA and can lead to cell mutations, cancer and birth defects.

**8.** When a heavy metal is placed in the mouth in the form of a metallic dental filling, a "battery effect" is created by the interaction of the metals in the filling and the saliva in the mouth, resulting in corrosion, which will ultimately have a damaging effect on the body.

**Nickel:** dental crowns, root canals, hydrogenated oils, inexpensive jewelry, batteries, cigarette smoke and stainless steel.

**Lead:** old paint, auto exhaust, insecticides, bullets, pewter ware, some hair colorings, tap water, batteries, pottery glazes, candle wicks and stained glass.

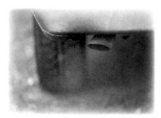

**Cadmium:** cigarettes, batteries, auto exhaust, pink dyes used in dentures, welding fumes, ceramic glazes, many art supplies, Teflon, fungicides and plastic.

**Copper:** some cooking utensils and plumbing, gold dental fillings and crowns, insecticides.

**Aluminum:** some drugs (including antacids), most baking powders, some cooking utensils, antiperspirants, cosmetics, foil, acid rain.

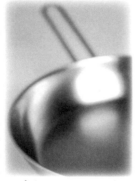

**Arsenic:** pesticides, smog, tobacco smoke, a by-product of metal ore smelting and coal-fired power plants, wood preservatives in lumber and playgrounds, green pigment used in toys, curtains, carpets and colored chalk.

**Platinum:** some dental gold, auto exhausts.

New sources of heavy metal exposure have been appearing with our evolving technology: "Electronic waste from discarded computers and other hardware is a main source of lead, mercury, cadmium and chromium."[29] There are numerous other sources of these (and other) metals, as well.

Although each metal produces its own set of unique symptoms at toxic levels, it is possible to generalize to some degree about common symptoms of heavy metal poisoning. Because heavy metals affect the human nervous system, the production of blood cells, the kidneys, the reproductive system and behavior, they may cause a wide variety of symptoms, including:

- Depression
- Irritability
- Numbness, tingling in the hands and feet
- Frequent urination
- Chronic fatigue
- Insomnia
- Poor circulation (cold hands and feet)
- Developmental retardation
- Kidney/liver damage
- Poor memory
- Temper tantrums
- Constipation and/or diarrhea
- Leg cramps
- Heartburn
- Skin rashes
- A metallic taste in the mouth
- Joint pain
- Rapid heart beat
- Excessive itching
- Tinnitus (ringing in the ears)
- Twitching of facial (and other) muscles
- Abdominal bloating
- Impaired immunity

Initially, symptoms tend to be mild, becoming more severe as toxicity increases. For example, "Memory loss, tremors, emotional instability (anxiety and irritability), insomnia and loss of appetite are all symptoms of mercury exposure. At moderate exposures, more significant mental disorders and motor disturbances, as well as kidney damage, are seen. More severe cases show constriction of vision, diminished hearing, speech disorders, shaky movements and unsteady gait."[30]

*"Approximately 8% of women had (mercury) concentrations higher than the US Environmental Protection Agency's recommended reference dose 95.8 microg/L, below which exposures are considered to be without adverse effects."*

*JAMA, 2004, April 2; 289(13): 1667-74*

The effects of heavy metals and pesticides may be synergistic — meaning that one magnifies the effects of the other. Mercury, for example, may impair detoxification, leading to higher levels of pesticides in those carrying heavy body burdens of mercury.

## Agricultural Toxins

Pesticides, of course, have long been used in commercial agriculture to protect crops from damage by insects. Unfortunately, residues of those pesticides remain on the harvested crop and ultimately end up in our bodies.

"The National Cancer Institute has repeatedly found that farmers have higher than average risks for several types of cancer affecting the blood (leukemia), brain and stomach. In general, they had a six times greater risk than non-farmers in developing cancer. Organic farming eliminated that risk.

Studies of farmers in the United States and elsewhere indicate they suffer from more depression or suicide than expected.

Children born to farmers who use fumigants and glyphosate or pesticide applicators were found to have more birth defects, especially if they were conceived in the spring and their offspring were also three times more likely to have some form of the attention deficit disorder (ADD). In addition, reports suggest they have a preponderance of female offspring."[31]

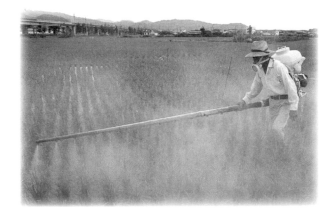

There is reason to believe (and hope) that ultimately, the pest problem on farms may be solved not through use of more potent pesticides, but through restoration of optimal mineral balance to the soil in which crops are grown. Just as we are coming to recognize the importance of the condition of the body's terrain (internal environment) to health, we are also becoming increasingly aware that the health of plants is dependent upon the condition of the soil (external terrain) in which they're grown.

Chemical "NPK" fertilizers (composed of nitrogen, phosphorous and potassium) have been widely used in agriculture for over a century. These fertilizers stimulate plant growth by returning just three minerals to the soil, which normally contains scores of minerals. In this way, the soil is made deficient in those critical trace minerals that are not re-supplied. This is similar to the situation we have created by "enriching" refined foods. After the refining process strips the food of dozens of critical nutrients, that food is "enriched" through the addition of just four nutrients (B1, B2, niacin and iron, in a synthetic form). Here again, a situation of imbalance is created, which makes the deficiency worse, rather than correcting it.

NPK fertilizer further affects the soil adversely by acidifying it, which has the net effect of killing off soil microorganisms whose job it is to break up and transmute, or change the nature of, minerals for use by the soil.[32] Without these critical microbes, soil minerals become locked up, and the health of the soil declines. Consequently, plants become malnourished, sick, and easy prey to insects. Here we may make another comparison: The over-acidified soil is like the human body that has become acidic as a result of eating a junk food diet. Such a body also becomes prey to "bugs" in the form of germs. The body that is acidic is toxic, for toxins are of an acid nature. By continually consuming commercial produce that is grown on nutrient-deficient soil and carries traces of toxic pesticides, we are further adding to the toxic burden carried by our bodies.

## Household Toxins

We tend to think of pollution as an outdoor phenomenon, when in fact, indoor environments are typically more polluted than outdoor ones, sometimes considerably more polluted. According to studies by the Environmental Protection Agency, "Indoor air levels of many pollutants may be 2 to 5 times, and on occasion more than 100 times higher than outdoor levels."[33] Our exposure to

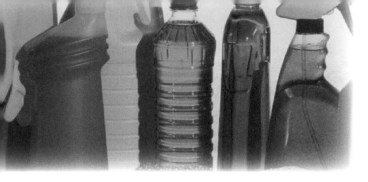

*Any chemical you can smell in the air makes its way into your bloodstream*

Dr. Sherry A. Rogers, Detoxify or Die, p.11

indoor pollutants has increased dramatically in recent years due largely to the construction of more tightly sealed, energy-efficient buildings in urban areas. These buildings are often poorly ventilated and constructed and furnished with synthetic materials. The escalating use of chemical-based consumer products inside such homes can be a recipe for disaster, especially in consideration of the fact that the average person spends 90% of his time indoors.[34]

Chemical contaminants in buildings contribute to "sick building syndrome," which is in reality "sick PERSON syndrome," a result of time spent in contaminated buildings. Such exposure can give rise to environmental illness, a growing problem today (and an area of specialization for some progressive physicians). Indoor chemical contaminants can be found in the air, the water supply, in building materials and in personal care or household items used by occupants of the building. Surprisingly, "Studies show that your risk of getting cancer from exposure to chemicals in the water and air in your home is greater than your risk from exposure to the same chemicals in a hazardous waste site."[35]

Sick Building Syndrome affects an estimated 40 million Americans,[36] though this may be an underestimate considering that most medical doctors are not trained in environmental medicine and are therefore not apt to correctly diagnose (and treat) environmental illness. Specialists, trained in Bau-Biologie, the science of building biology, and home inspection, can help to identify chemical contaminants and other stress factors (like electromagnetic radiation), that make up sick

## Common Sources of Indoor Pollution

**MORE INFO**

- Aerosol sprays
- Asbestos
- Bleach
- Carbon monoxide
- Carpets (synthetic), carpet adhesive
- Cleaning materials (including scouring pads and powders, oven cleaners, detergents, disinfectants, floor and furniture polish and wax and pot cleaners)
- Dry-cleaned clothing
- Gasoline
- Glue, rubber cement
- Heating systems or appliances: gas, oil, kerosene, propane or coal burning
- Insulation foam
- Lawn and garden chemicals
- Lead
- Mold
- Mothballs, moth crystals
- Newsprint
- Paint, paint remover
- Permanent markers/pens
- Personal care products
- Pesticides
- Plastics
- Plywood, particleboard
- Polyurethane, varnish
- Radon
- Room deodorizers
- Styrofoam (cups, plates, bowls, meat-wrapping materials)
- Synthetic fabrics
- Tap water
- Tobacco smoke
- Wood preservatives

Chart 2

building syndrome, as well as make recommendations for their remediation.

Up to 80% of the materials used in today's indoor environments are artificial.[37] Such materials "outgas" ("release or give off as a gas or vapor"[38]) dangerous chemicals that are inhaled by building occupants. Chart 2 lists items typically found in and around the home (or office) that may be harmful to occupants due to their chemical composition.

While space constraints won't allow for discussion of all household toxins, some are touched upon in the brief synopsis of selected indoor products/chemicals and their effects.

### Personal Care Products

Among the most damaging of the personal care products are those that are scented, for they affect not just the user but all with whom s/he is in contact. The strongest of the scented personal care products is cologne, or perfume but others may include deodorants, lotions, creams, bath salts, shampoo, cosmetics, soaps, body powders and oils.

"Up to 5000 different chemicals are used in various combinations in scented products, and 84% of these have had little or no human toxicology testing."[39]

Of the dozens of chemicals found in a single brand of cologne, three of the most damaging are the petrochemicals, alcohol and the penetrants. The penetrants (which give a fragrance its staying power) are the same ones used in insecticides.[40] This may be the reason that, to the chemically sensitive person, cologne smells like bug spray. Alcohol, used as a solvent (a substance that dissolves another substance) for these chemicals, is damaging to the fatty layer of cells and the protective covering of nerve cells in the body, having a solvent effect upon them as well.[41] Petrochemicals

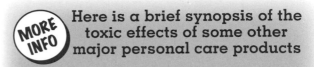

## Here is a brief synopsis of the toxic effects of some other major personal care products

- Cosmetics contain not only fragrances (with all their component chemicals), but also metal salts.
- Mascara and eyeliners may contain lead or coal tar dyes, which are also found in hair dyes.
- In addition, hair dyes contain aniline dyes, known to cause cancer in animals.
- Body powders made with talc can cause scarring of lung tissue when fine particles are inhaled.
- Most toothpaste and many mouthwashes on the market contain fluoride, promoted as a tooth-decay preventative. On the contrary, it is a highly toxic chemical, just a little less toxic than arsenic and a little more toxic than lead.[43] That's why there's a warning label on your toothpaste tube, telling you to call a poison control center if more than a pea-sized portion of the toothpaste is swallowed.
- Some shampoos and hair conditioners, hand lotions and hair colors contain a potentially dangerous antibacterial chemical called methylisothiazolinone (MIT). Animal studies showed that chronic exposure to this chemical had detrimental effects on the skin and nervous system.[44]
- Antibacterial hand soaps may also pose health risks due to the presence of triclosan. This chemical has been shown to inhibit bacterial growth, but also kill human cells.[45]
- Antibacterial ingredients may also be found in laundry detergents, dish soaps, toothpastes and mouthwashes. It's important to know that any substance that comes into contact with skin can be absorbed into the bloodstream and thus affect the entire body.

**When the National Institute of Occupational Safety and Health analyzed 2,983 chemicals used in personal care products, they found that:**

- 884 of the chemicals were toxic
- 314 caused biological mutations
- 218 caused reproductive complications
- 778 caused acute toxicity

Judith Berns, "The Cosmetic Cover-Up" as reported 5/7/04 in Health Alert Newsletter by Dr. James H. Martin

(waste products of the oil industry) feature prominently in cologne, for "95% of chemicals used in fragrances are synthetic compounds derived from petroleum, including many toxins and sensitizers that are capable of causing cancer, birth defects, central nervous system disorders and allergic reactions."[42] Toxins inhaled from the chemicals in cologne and other scented products go straight to the brain through the olfactory nerves.

# Some Ingredients to Avoid in Personal Care Products

- Propylene glycol
- Sodium lauryl sulfate
- Methyl or propyl paraben
- Imidazolidnyl urea
- Petrolatum
- Mineral oil
- Stearalkonium chloride
- Triethanolamine

It's also important to read labels, even though all ingredients are not always listed. If those that are listed are unknown to you and difficult to pronounce, chances are they are potentially toxic chemicals that are best avoided.

## Volatile Organic Compounds

VOCs (which include chemicals like acetate and ethanol) have been found to have toxic effects, even at low doses. Many are suspected carcinogens. These chemically unstable compounds vaporize (turn to gas) readily and may combine with other chemicals to create compounds that can cause toxic reactions when inhaled or absorbed through the skin. VOCs can be found in cologne and can be released by many other products as well: carpet adhesives, paints, varnishes, paint strippers and other solvents, wood preservatives, aerosol sprays, cleansers, degreasers and disinfectants, moth repellents, air fresheners, stored fuels, automotive products, hobby supplies, dry-cleaned clothing and cosmetics.

Known adverse health effects of VOCs include eye and respiratory tract irritation, headaches, dizziness, visual distortions, impaired memory, depression, kidney problems, liver damage, nausea, loss of coordination, migraines, wheezing, asthma and nervous system damage.[46]

## Formaldehyde

Formaldehyde is a widely used chemical, both for manufacturing building materials and a number of household products. Many of these materials contain formaldehyde-based glues, resins, preservatives and bonding agents. The chemical is also found in smoke, unvented fuel-burning appliances, paper goods, household cleaners and foam insulation. The most significant source of formaldehyde in the indoor environment is probably pressed wood products (particle board, plywood and fiberboard). The release of formaldehyde from these woods diminishes with the age of the wood, lowered temperature and lowered humidity in the environment.

On their website, the EPA acknowledges that formaldehyde may cause cancer, and they list the following additional health effects: eye, nose, and throat irritation; wheezing and coughing; fatigue; skin rash; and severe allergic reactions.[47] To these, we may add nausea, excessive thirst, nosebleeds, insomnia and disorientation.[48]

Many textile products have formaldehyde finishes. These include nylon and all polyester blends with permanent press fabrics. Synthetic carpets also contain formaldehyde, along with more than a dozen other hazardous chemicals (like xylene, benzene and toluene), chemicals that continue to outgas from the carpets for up to five years after installation.[49] The most dangerous stage of out-gassing is from four weeks to three months following installation. While carpets over five years old usually have stopped out-gassing, they

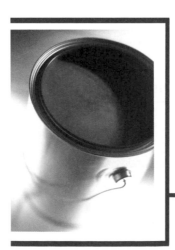

*According to the EPA, VOCs tend to be even higher (2-5 times) in indoor air than outdoor air, likely because they are present in so many household products.*

*www.mercola.com/fcgi/pf/2005/feb/19/ common_toxins.htm*

may then become breeding grounds for dust mites and mold.[50] Mold is a biological contaminant, rather than a chemical one, but it can give rise to damaging mycotoxins (fungal toxins).

## Mold

Mold is a "nonscientific term commonly used to describe just about any fungal growth."[51] If you had a mold problem in your home or office, you'd know it, right? Not necessarily. The sobering fact is that mold can grow and multiply in concealed areas of a building, such as air ducts, attics and wall cavities without producing obvious signs, but taking a toll upon your health nonetheless.

Fungi require moisture to grow, and most reproduce by releasing spores. Mold growth can be arrested by removing and replacing water-damaged building materials, cleaning exposed surfaces and controlling indoor humidity. However, if moldy materials are not *properly* removed (by professionals under "containment" conditions) and all affected surfaces thoroughly cleaned, other areas of the building may become contaminated with mold spores, spreading the problem. And, "Even if spores are no longer viable (alive), they can still contain allergens and mycotoxins that may affect health."[52]

There is a growing recognition today of the serious health threat that mold poses, as well as how problematic and costly its identification and remediation can be. For these reasons, some have dubbed mold "the new asbestos." Removal of both mold and asbestos is tricky business. If done improperly, the problem can be compounded. While asbestos litigation was yesterday's news, litigation regarding mold damage is in today's headlines: A Texas family was recently awarded $32.1 million after their insurance company failed to properly address their water damage and mold claim.

While allergic reaction to mold (experienced by one in three people)[53] is the most common health problem associated with exposure, the following symptoms (either alone or in combination) may also result:[54]

• Respiratory problems, such as wheezing and difficulty in breathing

• Nasal and sinus congestion
• Burning, watery, red eyes, blurred vision, light sensitivity
• Dry, hacking cough
• Sore throat
• Nose and throat irritation
• Shortness of breath
• Skin irritation
• Central nervous system problems (constant headaches, memory problems and mood changes)
• Aches and pains
• Possible fever

## Tap Water

People need water to survive. Unfortunately, the days are long gone when we could turn to our taps for a glass of pure, uncontaminated water.

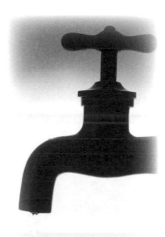

A minimal amount of drinking water contamination is to be expected as a result of natural processes; however, today's tap water, whether coming from municipal water supplies or private wells, from surface water or underground aquifers, is much more than minimally contaminated. The EPA only monitors 84 out of the 2,100 contaminants found in drinking water,[55] and a significant number of violations of the standards set for these 84 contaminants have been reported since the Safe Drinking Water Act was first enacted in 1974.[56]

Contaminants in drinking water may be either chemical or microbial. Microbial contaminants, such as viruses, bacteria, and parasites, come from human and animal waste. An outbreak of the microscopic parasite *cryptosporidium* in the Milwaukee water supply in 1993 killed over 100 people and sickened some 400,000.[57]

Chemical contaminants include pesticides, heavy metals, industrial waste, and even chemical by-products

# Some News About Tap Water

In December 2005 the Environmental Working Group released the results of a two-and-a-half year investigation of tap water served to communities across the country. In an analysis of more than 22 million tap water quality tests across the U.S., EWG detected over 300 types of contaminants in water served to the public. One hundred forty-one (141) of these detected chemicals are unregulated; meaning public health officials have no safety standards for them, even though millions drink them every day. Here is some of what they found:

83 agricultural pollutants, including pesticides and chemicals from fertilizers
59 contaminants linked to wastewater treatment plants
166 industrial chemicals from factory waste and consumer products
52 linked to cancer
41 linked to reproductive toxicity
36 linked to development toxicity
16 to immune system damage

The unregulated chemicals that pollute public tap water supplies include the gasoline additive MTBE; perchlorate from rocket fuel; industrial plasticizers and chemical pollutants from fuel combustion.

*Environmental Working Group*

created from the use of disinfecting agents. Bottled water can, and often does, contain contaminants.

The disinfecting agents most commonly used in US public water supplies are chlorine and chloramines, a combination of chlorine and ammonia. While chlorine effectively kills pathogens in the water, it can also have some undesirable effects upon our health. Some of these effects are a result of the chemicals that are formed when chlorine unites with organic matter to form *trihalomethanes* (ThMs), chemicals like chloroform, bromoform and carbon tetrachloride. ThMs have been

associated with atherosclerosis, and studies have shown a link between chlorination and increased incidences of bladder, colon and rectal cancer.[58] Chlorinated water also destroys much of our beneficial intestinal flora, needed to protect us from pathogens, and it can "destroy polyunsaturated fatty acids and vitamin E in the body, while generating toxins capable of free radical damage (oxidation)."[59]

Among the 84 pollutants monitored by the EPA is an array of pesticides, biological contaminants and other chemicals, including fluoride. This identification of fluoride as a pollutant may come as a shock to some, for we have been led to believe that it is an essential nutrient needed to prevent tooth decay, not a water pollutant. This is an inaccurate representation. The fact of the matter is that the EPA has set a Maximum Contaminant Level (an enforceable standard set for drinking water contaminants) for fluoride, substantiating that it is, indeed, a contaminant. To make matters worse, the form of fluoride used in water fluoridation programs is an industrial waste product. Over 90% of the fluoridated US municipal water supplies use *hydrofluorosilicic acid* as a fluoridating agent. This chemical is a highly toxic by-product of phosphate fertilizer production. Its presence in our drinking water is more about the corporate bottom line than about the claimed benefit of preventing tooth decay. The appalling aspect of this whole scenario is the adverse health affects that can result from fluoride exposure, even at the relatively low doses used in water fluoridation programs. These may include:

• Hyperactivity
• Learning disabilities
• Cancer
• Hypothyroidism
• Dental fluorosis (permanent discoloration of teeth) in children
• Arthritis
• Kidney disease
• Gastrointestinal disorders
• Birth defects
• Lowered immunity

Links to studies verifying the role of fluoride in these disorders and others may be found at http://www.slweb.org/bibliography.html, a website founded by Fluoride Action Network, a group formed in 2000 by scientists (including EPA scientists), dentists and environmentalists to educate the public on the toxicity of fluoride compounds and the health impacts of current fluoride exposures.

## Medical/Dental Toxins

We tend to make a distinction between "good" drugs (legal ones) and "bad" drugs (illegal ones), but the fact of the matter is that all drugs, even prescription and over-the-counter drugs, are toxic to some degree. While a medicine may effectively relieve an unpleasant symptom, the price paid in terms of potential side effects (both felt and unfelt) may be great. This fact is dramatically reflected in a lengthy and well-documented report compiled by three MDs and two PhDs based on their detailed analysis of medical literature and government health statistics and released in 2003 by the Nutritional Institute of America. In their paper, the team reports that the number of people who died in 2001 as a result of *iatrogenic* conditions (those brought on inadvertently by either medical treatment or diagnostic procedures) was *greater than* those who died in that same year of either heart disease or cancer,[60] the #1 and #2 leading causes of death in the US respectively. The numbers were as follows:

Deaths from cancer ............................................ 553,251
Deaths from heart disease .................................. 699,697
Deaths from iatrogenic conditions ..................... 783,936

The report further states that "Over 2.2 million people are injured every year by prescription drugs alone, and over 20 million unnecessary prescriptions for antibiotics are prescribed annually for viral infections."[61] Overuse of antibiotics has led to development of antibiotic-resistant organisms and has the net effect of reducing a patient's immune response because beneficial intestinal bacteria are eliminated.

Even drugs that are generally recognized as safe, such as aspirin, can cause serious side effects. Aspirin belongs to a class of drugs known as *non-steroidal anti-inflammatory drugs* (NSAIDs), which irritate the stomach lining, can cause ulcers and lead to leaky gut syndrome, thus permitting potentially damaging non-nutrient substances to gain access to the bloodstream. Steroids (such as cortisone and prednisone), also used to combat inflammation, may lead to deterioration of the intestinal lining as well.

Many medications adversely affect the body's detoxification organs, chief of which is the liver. Melissa Palmer, MD, tells us that there are over 1,000 drugs and chemicals that can cause injury to the liver,[62] thus compromising the body's detoxification capabilities.

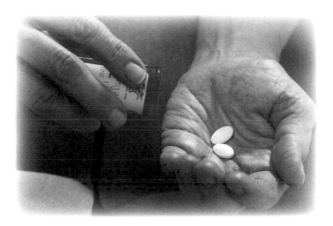

Dental materials and procedures also make a significant contribution to the body's toxic load, thereby creating disease conditions. An increasing number of progressive physicians are beginning to believe that a good portion of chronic disease has its roots in dental toxicity. While the best-known toxic dental material in use today is the controversial "silver" amalgam, which is over half mercury, many other potentially damaging metals (especially nickel and palladium) and non-metallic restorative materials are also in widespread use in dentistry today.

It is not only dental materials, but also some procedures, that are potentially toxic to the mouth and the body as a whole. The trauma to the jawbone caused by invasive dental procedures, such as root canal treatments and extractions done using routine protocol, has been associated with many problems. These include infection, poor blood flow (*ischemia*) to the jaw, and oral and systemic (whole-body) toxicity (bacterial toxins can travel throughout the body), as well as jawbone erosion (known popularly as "jawbone cavitations" and technically as "*osteonecrosis*").[63] Progressive dentists are continually seeking and finding safer ways to practice dentistry by refining standard techniques and by testing materials for *biocompatibility* — i.e., making sure that the materials used are safe for the individual patient.

# Chapter 2: Digestive Toxins

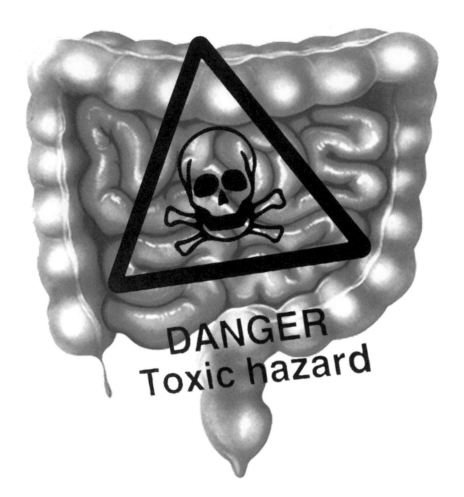

DANGER
Toxic hazard

## The definition of *autointoxication* is the 'poisoning, or the state of being poisoned, from toxic substances produced within the body.'

Chronic disease can be and often is the end result of poor digestion. Although environmental toxins are most certainly an important contributing factor, digestive toxins, which include those produced by harmful microbes in our gastrointestinal tracts, are an equally important, though often overlooked, source of disease in the body. These toxins can contribute to all manner of disease, not just gastrointestinal disorders (which affect the mouth, esophagus, stomach, intestines, liver, gallbladder and pancreas). Ultimately, poor digestion will encourage the advancement of age-related disorders and autoimmune diseases such as arthritis, fibromyalgia, chronic fatigue syndrome, food allergies and sensitivities. Such maladaptive responses to food are thought to develop when undigested food particles enter the circulatory system through the walls of the intestine (which has become weakened as a result of digestive toxins), and the body responds by launching an attack on them as though they were foreign invaders.

FACTS

## Digestive Disorders

- Digestive diseases affect 60 to 70 million people.
- 13% of all hospitalizations are for digestive disorders.
- Digestive disorders account for 50 million physician office visits per year.
- Digestive disorders cost $107 billion — $87 billion in direct medical costs and $20 billion in indirect costs each year.

http://www.healthsystem.virginia.edu/UVAHealth/adult_digest/index.cfm

When properly digested, carbohydrates are converted to glucose, protein to amino acids, and fats are broken down into glycerol and fatty acids. If these conversions are incomplete, food will not be in the proper form for our bodies to absorb. The food will therefore pass through the system undigested (or partially digested), producing toxins as a result. If the body is unable to promptly eliminate these toxins, either because the toxic load is too great and/or because detoxification channels (specific organs and systems discussed in the next section) are blocked, they will be retained and lead ultimately to chronic disease as chart 1 indicates).

## Factors Influencing Digestive Disturbance

Impaired or incomplete digestion can occur for a number of reasons, some of which are:

- Stress
- Processed food consumption
- Inadequate chewing, or drinking water or beverages with meals
- Improper food-combining
- Overeating

In the face of any of these factors, improperly digested food will ferment or putrefy (rot), giving rising to digestive toxins, listed on chart 1 as step 2, "Intestinal Toxemia."

**Stress**

When we experience stress in any form (physical, mental or emotional) energy (along with blood, enzymes and oxygen) is diverted away from the digestive organs so that it may be used to deal with the stress at hand. The result is a lowering of pancreatic enzyme production and inhibition of hydrochloric acid (HCl) or stomach acid production. Without vital enzymes and HCl, food is improperly digested, and toxins are produced.

The many environmental chemicals to which we're exposed daily in our food, air, water and consumer products constitute an ongoing physical stress, which can take a toll on the body's ability to properly digest food.

**Processed Food Consumption**

Not only is today's processed food loaded with chemicals (some 3,000+ food additives), but it is stripped of vital nutrients as well. During the refining process, dozens of essential nutrients, including trace minerals needed for carbohydrate combustion, are discarded when whole wheat and raw sugar are converted into white flour and white sugar. These refined carbohydrates are seriously deficient in many nutrients, including the minerals chromium, manganese, cobalt, copper, zinc and magnesium. When the body has exhausted its storehouses of these important minerals, it is no longer able to properly digest carbohydrates. Consequently, the partially digested carbohydrates (sugars and starches) will ferment (be converted into simple sugars and alcohol), providing fuel for yeast and bacteria and leading to indigestion and gas and bloating, which increases the toxic load of the body.

### Stages of Declining Health

1. Impaired Digestion
2. Intestinal Toxemia
3. Candida and Parasites
4. Imbalance of Gut Flora
5. Leaky Gut
6. Chronic Disease

Chart 1

Fiber, naturally found in whole grains, fruits and in vegetables, provides the bulk necessary to move food residue through the intestines. Unfortunately, this vital non-nutrient is also discarded in the refining process. Without fiber, food residue moves much more slowly through the digestive tract, sometimes more than twice as slowly as it should.[1] Such a prolonged *transit time* (of food through the gastrointestinal tract) can result in constipation and subsequent absorption of toxins from fecal material that has been retained and has putrefied. This absorption of toxins from within the digestive system is a form of self-poisoning, which has been referred to as *autointoxication*.

### Inadequate Chewing/Excess Fluid Intake with Meals

Carbohydrate digestion begins in the mouth when the enzyme *ptyalin* mixes with saliva and finely chewed food particles. When food is inadequately chewed, there is not enough time for this enzyme to become thoroughly mixed with saliva and food, and digestion becomes impaired. Digestive impairment can likewise result when large amounts of water or another beverage are consumed with meals, diluting digestive juices.

### Improper Food-Combining

Fruit, which is digested very rapidly when eaten alone, is often served as a dessert with foods that take longer to digest (starchy carbohydrates, fats and/or protein). This delays the movement of the fruit through the GI tract, causing it to ferment, which gives rise to production of inner toxins.

Eating heavy proteins (like meat) at the same meal with starchy carbohydrates (like grains or potatoes) can also lead to digestive stress, inadequate digestion and subsequent generation of digestive toxins. This is because proteins require an acid digestive secretion, while carbohydrates call for an alkaline secretion. Acid and alkaline solutions cancel each other out, resulting in inadequate digestion of either the protein or the starch, and subsequent generation of digestive toxins.

### Overeating

Eating too much, even of the best-quality food, will stress the digestive organs by making heavy demands upon them and depleting them of energy. Also, if the food

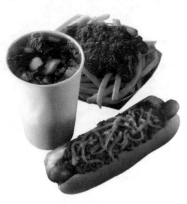

consumed is cooked, it will not contain *food enzymes*, found only in raw foods, and the body will become enzyme depleted, further compromising digestive capability. Animal studies have correlated overeating with a reduced life span.[2]

## Results of Digestive Disturbance

While stress is listed above as a separate contributing factor in poor digestion, the other factors — consumption of processed food, inadequate chewing, drinking liquids with meals, combining foods improperly and overeating — may all be viewed as stressors (types of stress) that can adversely affect digestion by producing any of the following consequences:

- Reduced HCl production
- Reduced enzyme production
- Imbalanced intestinal pH
- Food sensitivities

### Reduced HCl Production

HCl is a strong acid produced in the stomach. Among its other functions, it helps break down protein into amino acids and destroys harmful microbes that may be present in food. The presence of HCl also signals the production of pepsin, a protein-splitting enzyme, which further assures the complete break down of protein components.

It is a common misconception that too much HCl causes such GI disorders as indigestion, heartburn and ulcers. The truth is these disorders may be present in the face of either too much or too little stomach acid. Nonetheless, indigestion and heartburn are often treated medically with antacids without any attempt to actually measure HCl levels. While this may result in temporary relief of symptoms, in the long run it may make matters worse, particularly if an under-production of HCl is the actual cause of the condition, which is often the case. When drugs are used to inhibit HCl production, stomach becomes alkaline, and the body responds by producing more acid, which is then treated with more antacids, creating a vicious cycle. The net result will be exhaustion of the acid-producing cells in the stomach and its subsequent inability to continue producing HCl.

### Reduced Enzyme Production (Pancreatic Insufficiency)

The pancreas secretes enzymes called *protease* to break down protein, *amylase* to break down carbohydrates, and *lipase* for fat digestion. When these secretions are inadequate (a condition known as *pancreatic insufficiency*), digestion is incomplete, and the result is likely to be development of such symptoms as gas, indigestion, bloating and food sensitivities. Pancreatic insufficiency may be caused by stress, nutrient deficiency, over-consumption of cooked food, toxic exposure, aging, drugs, infection or low HCl production.

The enzymes produced by the pancreas are known collectively as *digestive* enzymes. Other classes of enzymes are metabolic (which run and heal the body) and *food* enzymes, found naturally in uncooked food. When cooked foods are eaten exclusively, no food enzymes are supplied, putting an extra load on the body's digestive enzymes. The body may, in turn, redirect metabolic enzymes to help with digestion, making them unavailable to do their normal job of healing.

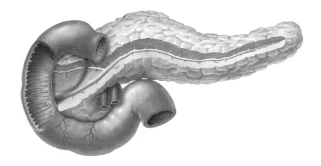

### Imbalances Intestinal pH

PH is a measurement of acidity/alkalinity. Different parts of the GI tract have different pH levels, making them either acid (low pH) or alkaline (high pH). In a healthy body, the mouth is alkaline, the stomach is

acid, the small intestine alkaline and the colon acid. These pH conditions must be maintained for complete digestion to occur and optimal health to be achieved and maintained. An imbalance in pH may result from inadequate HCl (possibly the result of using antacids), which makes the stomach alkaline, or from pancreatic insufficiency, which can make the small intestine acid.

### Food Sensitivities

A food sensitivity is technically different than an allergy in that it involves a delayed response to the *allergen* (allergic food), rather than an immediate one, and involves production of different *antibodies*, (chemical bullets used to attack foreign invaders). However, in both instances, a maladaptive response to food or food components is involved, a response that is thought to be autoimmune in nature. Such a response, as noted, involves the inappropriate launching of an immune attack upon undigested or partially digested food particles that have entered the bloodstream due to increased permeability of the intestinal lining. This condition, known as *leaky gut syndrome* (shown as step 5 in chart 1), is discussed below.

## Intestinal Toxemia and Its Consequences

Intestinal toxemia (poisoning of the intestines) is the immediate consequence of impaired digestion brought on by the factors described above. If we fail to digest our food, intestinal bacteria will digest it, leaving behind their waste products to poison our bodies. These bacterial toxins are extremely potent. Some of the most damaging of the 78 known types are skatoles, indoles, phenols, alcohol, ammonia, acetaldehyde and formaldehyde.

Intestinal toxins such as these can produce cell-damaging *free radicals*, molecules with unpaired electrons that steal electrons from cell membranes, wreaking biochemical havoc in the body. Free radical damage has been associated with the aging process and with chronic disease. Antioxidant nutrients, such as vitamins A, C and E and the minerals selenium and zinc, enable us to buffer free radicals, preventing them from inflicting damage up to a point. Once we have become deficient in the antioxidant nutrients and/or our toxic load becomes too great, free radicals go unchecked. At this point, opportunistic organisms such as viruses, bacteria, parasites and fungi multiply (step

3 in chart 1). Their toxic waste products will ultimately overwhelm the body's defenses, allowing these microorganisms to continue multiplying freely. This can cause such symptoms as gas, bloating, constipation, diarrhea, skin disorders, brain fog, chronic fatigue, irritable bowel syndrome, joint pain and muscle pain.

At this point, it's worth noting that not all gut bacteria are harmful. On the contrary, many of them (ideally about 80%) are beneficial. "Friendly" intestinal bacteria (also known as *flora* or probiotics) are vital to our very survival, for they perform numerous critical functions. Among other things, they:

- Help to maintain normal cell growth and regeneration
- Maintain normal, healthy stool consistency
- Maintain a balanced intestinal pH
- Produce vitamin K and the B vitamins
- Maintain normal bowel function, tone and condition
- Produce enzymes that aid in the digestion of lactose[3]

The ideal ratio of "good" to harmful bacteria is about 80% to 20%. When this ratio becomes distorted due to factors enumerated in chart 2, conditions are ripe for such opportunistic organisms as *Candida albicans* to proliferate or overgrow. Under normal circumstances, moderate amounts of this yeast/fungus are present in the digestive tract and cause no harm, as they are in balance with the trillions of bacteria that also reside there. The desired candida/bacteria ratio becomes disturbed, however, if:

- The immune system is not functioning normally.
- The ratio of "good/neutral" to "bad" intestinal bacteria is disturbed.
- The pH of the colon is incorrect (alkaline rather than acid)

We've already seen how immunity becomes impaired as a result of intestinal toxemia giving rise to free radicals and multiplication of microorganisms such as candida. Once candida proliferates, taking on a fungal form, it causes sugar cravings since fungi must have sugar to survive. Giving in to these cravings will feed candida and further depress immunity. An overconsumption of sugar and other refined carbohydrates can also give rise to a proliferation of bad bacteria in the gut, as can many other factors (shown in chart 2).

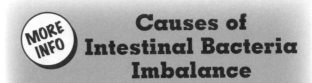

# Causes of Intestinal Bacteria Imbalance

- Antibiotic use
- Refined carbohydrates
- Birth control pills
- Poor digestion/elimination
- Stress
- Low-fiber diet
- Steroid drug use
- X-ray/radiation therapy
- Chlorinated water
- Mercury toxicity
- Pollution

Chart 2

Once the normal ratio of good bacteria (or flora) to bad bacteria is disturbed (step 4 in chart 1), immune impairment increases, and digestion of food and absorption of its nutrients become impaired. The bowel tends to become sluggish, causing retention of toxins. A sluggish bowel can also result when the pH of the colon is incorrect. Normally acidic, the pH of the colon may become too alkaline as pH disturbances occur elsewhere in the GI tract. Candida secretes acid, which can change the pH of the small intestine (normally alkaline) and cause wear to its protective mucous lining. Further damage to this lining is caused when candida's long roots (*rhizoids*) puncture it. The resulting increased intestinal permeability is known as *leaky gut syndrome* (step 5 in chart 1). This condition permits the entry of candida and its toxins, along with other non-nutrient substances and allergy-causing undigested food particles, into the bloodstream.

Once pathogens and toxins have entered the bloodstream, they are carried first to the liver and then to other organs throughout the body. If the liver's detoxification ability is impaired due to nutritional deficiency and/or toxic overload, these toxins will be stored (often in the weakest areas of the body) and can initiate chronic disease (step 6 in chart 1). Some of the disorders that may result from toxicity are discussed at the end of the next chapter.

**Digestive Tract**

**Bloodstream**

**Liver**

**Systemic Toxicity**

**Veins are colon's link to bloodstream**

# Chapter 3: **Channels of Elimination**

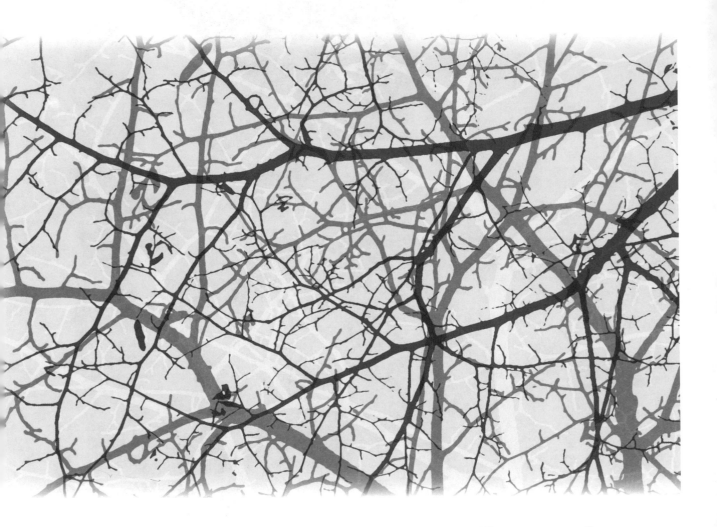

# Human blood travels 60,000 miles per day on it's journey through the body.

The body has seven channels of elimination: the blood, the lymphatic system, and five organs — the colon, kidneys, lungs, skin and liver. All have a unique role to play in getting rid of toxins, and all must be functioning optimally for effective total body detoxification. The lungs go into action when we breathe, eliminating toxic waste from the body in the form of carbon dioxide during the exhalation cycle. When we perspire, toxins come out through the skin as we sweat.

Two separate circulatory systems, containing blood and lymph respectively, play an important role in the detoxification process. The blood that flows through the vessels of the *vascular* (blood circulatory) system carries both oxygen and nutrients to the cells. That oxygen is essential for oxidizing or burning off toxins. Blood circulation is vital for transporting toxins to organs of elimination. Conversely, the bloodstream may also serve as a distribution line for toxins when they enter it through a leaky gut. Cellular health depends upon a clean bloodstream. The other circulatory system is the lymphatic system, which is the body's pumping system to eliminate poisons from cells. Unlike the vascular system that has an actual pump (the heart), the lymphatic system has no real pump and must depend solely upon the pumping action of our movement via exercise and deep breathing. The lymphatic system is an important focus of immune system activity in the body. Lymph fluid contains white blood cells (immune cells). Lymph nodes (bean-shaped structures along lymphatic capillaries, concentrated in groin, armpits, neck and abdomen), serve as depositories for these immune cells and as centers for disposing of the remains of dead microorganisms.

Toxins from the digestive system and the liver are excreted in the form of bowel eliminations from the colon. Water-soluble toxins from the liver are excreted in the urine from the kidneys (the organ that regulates the composition of the blood) via the bladder. Both bowel and kidney eliminations contain toxins that were first acted upon by the liver in a two-step detoxification process described in the following discussion of the liver.

## The Liver

Toxins that enter the body from the intestinal tract are transported to the liver, the largest and most active organ in the body and our primary detoxification channel. We cannot live without a <u>liver</u>. It is constantly working to cleanse and filter the 100 gallons of blood that flow through it every day. As our chief cleansing organ, the liver breaks down or transforms both inner and outer toxins so that they can be safely eliminated from the body. It contains special cells called *Kupffer cells* that ingest and break down toxic matter. The liver is also responsible for removing dead cells, the remains of microorganisms and other debris from the bloodstream.

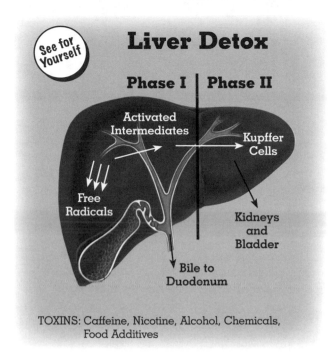

TOXINS: Caffeine, Nicotine, Alcohol, Chemicals, Food Additives

In addition to detoxification, the liver performs some 500 other bodily functions. It plays a role in blood sugar regulation, metabolizes fats, carbohydrates and proteins, synthesizes blood-clotting factors and manufactures *bile*. About one quart of this fat-emulsifying substance is produced every day and stored temporarily in the gallbladder, to be released when ingested dietary fat makes its way to the intestines. In addition to emulsifying fat, bile also lubricates the intestines, assists in absorption of fat-soluble vitamins and promotes *peristalsis* (wave-like muscular movements in the intestines). Also, some toxins are carried out of the body in the bile through the stool.

Inside the liver cells all toxic substances are broken down (or *biotransformed*) by two complex mechanisms known as Phase 1 and Phase 2 detoxification pathways. These pathways require specific nutrients to function properly. When the needed nutrients are adequately supplied, fat-soluble toxins (those that dissolve only in fat, not water and are commonly stored in our fatty tissues and cell membranes) are converted into a more easily excreted water-soluble form. The excretion routes are the kidneys (through urine) and bowels (through feces).

Phase 1 is known technically as the "cytochrome P-450 mixed function oxidase enzyme pathway'" (P-450 for short). This pathway contains dozens of enzymes, each of which specializes in detoxification of certain chemicals. With a deficiency of any of these enzymes, the P-450 system becomes impaired, which can result in toxins being stored rather than eliminated. Phase 1 enzymes will either directly neutralize a toxin for excretion through the bile or urine or convert that toxin into a more active form that is passed on for further processing in Phase 2.

The process of preparing toxins for Phase 2 detoxification (so that they may ultimately be rendered harmless) also produces free radicals, which can damage liver cells. These free radicals are produced in Phase 1 as fat-soluble toxins are being converted into new substances called *active intermediaries*. Active intermediaries can actually do more damage than the original toxins if not promptly eliminated from the body. Antioxidant nutrients will offset free radical damage, but such damage can be pronounced when free radical-fighting antioxidants are in short supply, especially if toxic exposure is significant. High levels of free radicals can result from disruption of the Phase 1 detoxification process by exposure to excessive amounts of such toxins as caffeine, alcohol, dioxin, paint fumes, sulfonamides, exhaust fumes, barbiturates and organophosphorus pesticides.[1]

The Phase 2 liver detoxification process is called the *conjugation* pathway. The conjugation process involves a conversion of the intermediaries produced in Phase 1 with another substance, commonly a sulfur-bearing amino acid (such as taurine or cysteine), which converts the intermediary into a water-soluble form. That toxin can then be excreted from the body through bile or urine (via colon or kidneys).

When Phase 1 reactions are more active than Phase 2 reactions, the accumulation of active intermediaries can lead to tissue damage and disease. Over a period of time, such a pattern can result in the development of chemical sensitivities, where people are over-sensitive to environmental toxins. If either Phase 1 or Phase 2, or both, become overloaded, toxins will accumulate in the body, especially in fatty tissue, where they may remain for life. The brain and endocrine (hormonal) glands are common sites for toxin accumulation, which can result in brain dysfunction and hormonal imbalances,[2] giving rise to a number of cognitive, emotional and physical problems.

## Liver Stress

The barrage of toxins to which we're exposed today, virtually everywhere on the planet, but especially in industrialized societies, is unprecedented in history. This excessive exposure means that our livers are under more stress than the livers of our parents and grandparents. Such stress increases our nutritional needs, but sadly, today's standard diet of refined, enriched, preserved, irradiated, genetically modified, pasteurized, homogenized, hydrogenated, and otherwise processed foods doesn't begin to meet our increased nutritional needs. In fact, today's foods are actually less nutritious than their counterparts of yesteryear, owing largely to methods employed by modern agribusiness to increase agricultural yield and shelf life at the expense of nutrient content and consumer health. The combined stresses of nutrient depletion and toxicity lead to liver stress, dysfunction and ultimately disease.

The daily toll that is taken on our liver by undernutrition (often coupled with overeating) and toxic overload is not immediately apparent. In fact, it is possible for a person whose liver function is compromised by as much as 70% to have no symptoms, nor any clinical sign of liver impairment.[3] While people with hepatitis or cirrhosis have obvious liver disease, it is not widely recognized that those with such chronic diseases as cancer, diabetes, arthritis and osteoporosis generally have

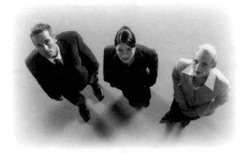

*In my experience of over 20 years of clinical medicine, I have found that approximately one in every three persons has a dysfunctional liver.*

Sandra Cabot, MD, author of the Liver Cleansing Book

## Some Signs of Liver Dysfunction

- Coated tongue
- Skin rashes
- Itchy skin
- Excessive sweating
- Offensive body odor
- Dark circles under eyes
- Yellow discoloration of eyes
- Liver spots (brown spots on skin)
- Acne rosacea (red pimples around nose, cheeks and chin)
- Red palms and soles, which may also be itchy and inflamed
- Flushed facial appearance or excessive facial blood vessels[4]

poor liver function as well. Liver dysfunction can give rise to virtually any disorder, for it adversely affects the digestive, immune, endocrine, circulatory and nervous systems in a variety of ways.

When the liver is toxic and congested, fats are not metabolized properly. This can lead to an obstruction of blood vessels, high blood pressure, heart attacks and stroke. As fat builds up in the liver and other organs, the metabolism (conversion of food to energy) slows down, resulting in weight gain (especially in the belly) and the appearance of unsightly cellulite deposits.

Because a toxic liver is not filtering properly, it is unable to rid the bloodstream of undigested food particles that have arrived there via a leaky gut, giving rise to an autoimmune response. Thus, a person with a toxic liver will be prone to allergies (the net result of this process), slowly becoming allergic to virtually everything if steps aren't taken to detoxify the liver.

Blood sugar problems (both hypoglycemia and adult onset diabetes) are common in those with a fatty liver; as are depression, brain fog, indigestion, constipation, bloating, recurrent infections, chronic fatigue, fibromyalgia and more.

Since the liver is our first line of defense against toxins, when it is overworked, an extra load is placed upon our other organs of detoxification. That extra load is passed from one organ system to another until either detoxification occurs, enabling the body to regain balance, or degeneration sets in. Many years ago, the late master herbalist Stuart Wheelwright dubbed this domino effect the *toxic stress cycle*. What follows is a brief description of that cycle.

## The Toxic Stress Cycle

The digestive system is the starting point in the toxic stress cycle. When food is not properly digested, toxins are produced in the intestine. These toxins then travel within the blood from the intestine to the liver via the portal vein. The liver, stressed and congested from overload (and nutrient deficiency), is incapable of managing these toxins and so they are passed out of the liver, through the hepatic veins into the systemic circulation. A portion of the toxins may be secreted through the skin, kidneys and lungs as the toxin-laden blood reaches these organs. The remainder is stored in the bones, hair, muscles (both skeletal and heart muscle), lymphatic tissue or fatty tissue. These stored toxins greatly affect energy production and hormone and enzyme functions that control free radical production. When free radicals dominate and key cellular functions (energy, hormone and enzyme production) become impaired, the body suffers and gradually becomes diseased.

Water retention may occur, as well as pH imbalance and long-term metabolic disturbances, when the kidneys are unable to perform their job of filtering the blood. If the next organ in line, the lungs, is unable to get rid of the toxins, they remain in the blood, interfering with oxygen absorption. Insufficient oxygen means insufficient metabolizing of sugars, fats and proteins. This, according to Wheelwright's toxic stress cycle,[5] leads to lymphatic congestion and a final shuffling of toxins to organs not designed for detoxification. The result may be heart problems, muscle pain and stiffness, spinal misalignments, impaired nerve supply to the brain and other organs and an energetic and nutritional depletion of the endocrine (hormonal) system. The net result is an underproduction of pancreatic enzymes needed for digestion, which brings us back full circle to the poor digestion where the problem began in the first place.

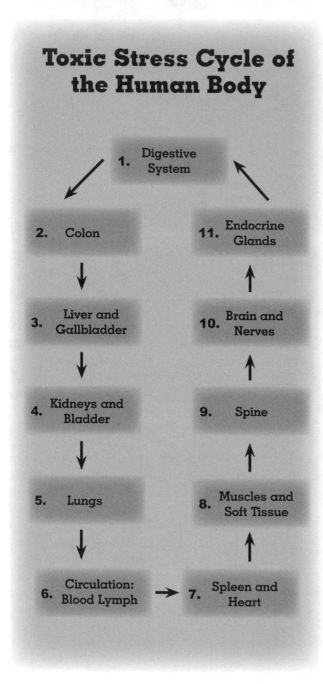

# Toxic Stress Cycle of the Human Body

1. Digestive System
2. Colon
3. Liver and Gallbladder
4. Kidneys and Bladder
5. Lungs
6. Circulation: Blood Lymph
7. Spleen and Heart
8. Muscles and Soft Tissue
9. Spine
10. Brain and Nerves
11. Endocrine Glands

## Toxicity and Chronic Disease

The net result of the toxic stress cycle is continuous digestive stress, which leads to retention of toxins and development of chronic disease, for as toxins are retained they cause irritation and inflammation to tissues. Most diseases have a strong toxicity component, the name of the disease often serving as an indicator of the location of the toxicity or the type of tissue affected by it. For example, in coronary (heart) disease, we would find toxins settling primarily in the coronary vessels; in joint diseases like arthritis and muscular problems like fibromyalgia, these toxins would be concentrated in the muscles or joints; toxic settlements in the pancreas and liver can play a significant role in diabetes and other blood sugar problems. As has been noted, toxins tend to settle in organs of greatest weakness.

Sometimes the toxic accumulation, rather than being found at the site of the symptom, occurs in an area that is energetically related, or located on the same energy pathway. For example, a heart problem may have its origin in a disturbance at a tooth site that shares the same acupuncture meridian (energy channel) as the affected organ. The heart problem could be the result of inflammation, infection or other problem in a wisdom tooth, as wisdom teeth cross the heart meridian. This would be an example of a focal condition. Focal infections can also cause problems in distant organs when toxins travel via the bloodstream or the lymphatic capillaries to other areas of the body.

## What follows is a very brief summary of how toxicity can contribute to some of today's most prevalent disorders

### Heart Disease

A major cause of heart disease is damage by free radicals to the individual cells within the arteries. Certain chemicals and heavy metals may play a major role, for they increase both the number and the activity of free radicals in the body. Many toxic metals — mercury, arsenic, aluminum, cadmium and lead — have been linked to heart disease. As noted, toxic metals will often displace nutrient minerals, creating a deficiency. Nutrient imbalances that have been associated with heart disease include copper imbalance, magnesium deficiency, fluoride toxicity and deficiencies of vitamin C and the amino acids proline and lysine. Matthias Rath, MD has demonstrated the beneficial effect of providing these last three nutrients to support collagen (connective tissue) production, heal artery walls and reverse the build-up of plaque.[6] Vitamin C additionally helps to detoxify the body, addressing a primary cause of the condition.

## High Cholesterol and Triglycerides

While these blood factors have been associated with cardiovascular diseases (such as heart attacks, stroke and high blood pressure), there is evidence that they are the result, rather than the cause, of such disorders. The body uses cholesterol and related metabolic products to attempt repair of structural weakness in the artery walls,[7] such weakness being the result of toxic damage and nutrient deficiency. Cholesterol levels, moreover, are controlled by the liver, whose regulatory ability is compromised when the body is overloaded with toxins.

## Arthritis

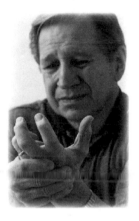

This painful joint disease stems from degeneration of connective tissue. It has been acknowledged that toxins play a major role in a process (known as the *inflammatory cascade*) that results in production of a class of inflammatory compounds (*leukotrienes*) that trigger white blood cells to release oxidants (free radicals), which attack tissue, resulting in inflammation or irritation.[8] Degeneration is the long-term effect of this process. In a paper published in the *JACA Journal of the American Chiropractic Association* in September of 1993, Dr. Alan H. Pressman states, "There is now a considerable body of evidence indicating that many ... degenerative joint disease conditions are associated with permeable [leaky] gut, liver detoxification pathways and activation of the pain-producing inflammatory cascade."[9] Impaired blood circulation appears to also play a role in arthritis. When there is no blood supply to the cartilage in joint spaces, then there is no direct supply of nutrients. Therefore, cartilage must absorb nutrients from the surrounding fluid. Impaired blood circulation results in lack of nutrients and oxygen in joint spaces and inability to clear toxic deposits.

## Fibromyalgia

This chronic pain syndrome affects the musculoskeletal system and expresses as fatigue and soreness in specific multiple points in the body. The symptom of fatigue is also commonly experienced with chemical sensitivities and allergies, both of which have a connection to toxic overload and may be part of the clinical picture in those suffering with fibromyalgia. As discussed, sensitivities and allergies often result from leaky gut syndrome, which allows passage of undigested proteins through the gut lining into the bloodstream, triggering an immune response. Given this scenario, it is not surprising that gastrointestinal disturbances are also common with fibromyalgia and that the symptoms of the disease are similar to those of bowel toxicity. The above quote by Dr. Pressman (in the "Arthritis" paragraph) also applies to fibromyalgia: it is a condition that involves not only leaky gut (a hyperpermeable gut) but also the pain-producing inflammatory cascade and blockage of liver detoxification pathways. While the medical cause of fibromyalgia is officially "unknown," it has been linked not only with leaky gut and liver toxicity, but also with chemical/pesticide exposure, nutrient deficiency, heavy metal toxicity, candida overgrowth and weakened immunity.

## Chronic Fatigue Syndrome

Not surprisingly, the dominant symptom in CFS (as in many other chronic conditions) is fatigue. This lack of energy is experienced right down to the cellular level as a result of toxic build-up and nutrient deficiency. These two conditions go hand in hand, for in the face of toxicity, nutrients cannot be properly utilized, even if abundantly supplied. Conversely, when vital nutrients are undersupplied, the functioning of organs and systems, including those involved in detoxification, is impaired, allowing toxins to accumulate. The metabolism of food is its conversion into energy. When metabolism slows down due to toxic overload, energy production is reduced, and we feel tired. With chronic fatigue comes adrenal insufficiency. Exhausted adrenals are unable to produce sufficient hormones, and this leaves the body vulnerable to all types of infection, including bacteria, yeast and parasites. These microorganisms, in turn, produce toxins, adding to the body's toxic load and increasing the fatigue.

## Obesity

When toxins accumulate, metabolism slows down, and the body's ability to convert food to energy diminishes. Water will often be retained in an effort to dilute these toxins. This results in heavy, waterlogged tissues and extra body weight. The body also retains fat in an

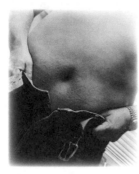

effort to dilute and store oil-soluble toxins, resulting in more weight gain. As toxicity increases in our environment, obesity becomes a growing problem. The two are related, though you'd never know it to read most diet books, which focus instead on counting calories or carbohydrates. Detoxification is an overlooked weight management tool, as well as the key to healthful living. A healthy liver is able to process fats, but a clogged one is not. Consequently, fatty deposits can accumulate, causing overweight conditions and increasing the risk of developing of cardiovascular disease.

## Depression

Depression, anxiety and other negative emotional states can actually result from nutrient deficiency and toxic accumulation in the body. For the brain, like any other organ, must be supplied with an abundance of nutrients and oxygen through the bloodstream. And, like any other organ, it can suffer from the effects of toxic build-up when these are inadequately supplied. Nature has created a "blood-brain barrier" whose job it is to prevent toxins from gaining access to the brain. Fat-soluble molecules, such as ethanol and caffeine, can penetrate the barrier relatively easily through the fatty membranes of its cells, while water-soluble molecules,

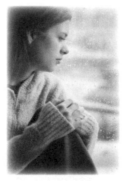

such as sodium and potassium, cannot cross it under normal circumstances. Unfortunately, some heavy metals (such as lead and mercury) and some harmful chemicals (such as fluoride) have the ability to cross this barrier. Fluoride forms bonds with most other substances (some toxic ones included), and in so doing, may help escort them across the blood-brain barrier, as well. Toxins that can damage the brain and nervous system are known as neurotoxins. These toxins can alter brain function, adversely affecting our moods and mental abilities.

## Cancer

A large and growing number of environmental toxins

## Some Cancer-Causing Substances and the Organs They Affect

| | |
|---|---|
| Formaldehyde | brain, kidneys, skin |
| Nickel | sinuses, breasts, reproductive organs, pancreas |
| Plastics | lungs, stomach, bladder |
| Pesticides | lungs, esophagus |
| Chlorinated solvents | lungs |
| Fiberglass | leukemia (bone marrow), lungs |
| Benzene | leukemia (bone marrow) |
| Tar | skin, sinuses |
| Asbestos | lungs |

From *Surviving the Toxic Crisis* by Dr. William R. Kellas and Dr. Andrea Sharon Dworkin

have been identified as carcinogenic (cancer-causing). The chart above shows some common carcinogens and the area/s of the body they commonly affect:

It is not just environmental toxins that can give rise to cancer. Internally produced toxins can do so as well. Waste products from microorganisms produce dozens of extremely potent toxins. These inner toxins can cause cell damage through free radical production, a process that can lead ultimately to cancer.

All of these toxins both inner and outer irritate weakened organs when the liver is unable to detoxify them adequately due to dysfunction, toxic overload or both. The net result of this irritation can be the development of cancerous tissue. A properly functioning liver is therefore your first line of defense against toxicity.

## Diabetes

Diabetes is a blood sugar disorder involving insufficient insulin. There are two major types: Type 1 (also known as insulin-dependent diabetes or juvenile diabetes) and Type 2 (non-insulin-dependent diabetes mellitus or adult-onset diabetes). Type 2 affects the vast majority (90%-95%) of diabetes sufferers. Type 1 is an autoimmune disease in which the body's immune system attacks and destroys the insulin-producing cells in the pancreas. Type 2 diabetics do produce insulin, but they either do so in insufficient amounts to fuel the cells or they experience "insulin resistance." In this instance, something is preventing the insulin from getting to the cells. This something is thought, by some experts, to be toxicity, while others attribute it to a genetic defect. Officially, however, the cause of insulin resistance is unknown, though it is known that the condition is aggravated by obesity and physical inactivity. The role of diet in blood sugar disorders is extremely important, for over-consumption of carbohydrates will cause an abrupt rise in blood sugar, demanding an immediate insulin response. Over a period of time, the pancreas becomes over-stimulated, initially producing too much insulin (a condition known as low blood sugar or hypoglycemia). Eventually, the organ may become sluggish, at which time insulin secretion decreases and diabetes (hyperglycemia) develops. The pancreas also produces digestive enzymes. Toxic damage to it may thus adversely affect both insulin and enzyme production.

The liver, as well as the pancreas, plays a role in regulating blood sugar, for it stores extra glucose (as glycogen) for future use. Toxic damage to the liver can prevent it from properly carrying out this function.

## Gastrointestinal Disorders

GI problems are those that affect any area of the GI tract (mouth, esophagus, stomach, small intestine and large intestine) and organs involved in digestion (pancreas and liver). These conditions, their causes and treatments (both medical and alternative), are described at length in *Gut Solutions*.

Many GI problems stem from *intestinal toxemia*, poisoning of the intestines, which occurs when the bacteria present act upon undigested food particles. This interaction produces toxic chemicals and gases (resulting in symptoms of gas and bloating). These toxins, in turn, can damage the mucosal lining, resulting in increased intestinal permeability (leaky gut). The net

result is that toxins are then able to spread throughout the body via the bloodstream, causing problems at distant sites. A few of the most prevalent GI disorders are discussed below with regard to their relationship to toxicity.

## Constipation

Constipation occurs when bowel transit time is reduced, meaning that food passes more slowly than normal through the GI tract. This is often due to insufficient intake of fiber-rich foods (fruits and vegetables) needed to increase peristalsis, the muscular movement that helps move food residue through the digestive tract. Slow transit time can lead to a build-up of toxic material on the intestinal walls, resulting in reduced nutrient absorption and subsequent lack of energy.

## Diarrhea

Diarrhea occurs when bowel transit time is too rapid. When stools are eliminated from the body to quickly, there is insufficient time for water from it to be re absorbed into the body. The result is that the stools retain water and become runny. Rapid bowel transit time is often brought on by toxic irritation. Acute diarrhea resulting from food poisoning is an example of this. Tissues are irritated by the toxic food and so the body tries to eliminate it as quickly as possible.

## Irritable Bowel Syndrome

This "functional" bowel disorder, characterized by abdominal pain, altered bowel habits, a sense of incomplete bowel elimination, and bloating, exhibits no structural abnormalities, leading to the inaccurate notion held by some that it is a psychological problem, not a physical one. Food sensitivities, especially lactose intolerance, appear to play a central role in IBS and occur in one-half to two-thirds of those afflicted. The most common allergens are dairy products and grains (especially wheat and corn). Food sensitivities, as has been noted, can develop as a consequence of leaky gut syndrome, where undigested proteins and toxins enter the bloodstream through the mucosal lining of the intestine, triggering an immune response.

## Gallstones

Among the causes of gallstones is over-production of cholesterol or under-production of bile by the liver. When either occurs, cholesterol crystals can precipitate out of solution and form one type of gallstone, the cholesterol stone. The liver's inability to maintain proper levels of cholesterol and bile, thus triggering stone formation, is often due to toxic overload. A toxic liver ultimately becomes inefficient in performing its many critical functions.

**Peptic Ulcers**

In recent years, it has been established that the bacterium *H. pylori* plays a major contributing role in ulcer formation. Other significant factors include heavy smoking, alcohol consumption, non-steroidal anti-inflammatory drugs (such as aspirin), caffeine-containing beverages, steroid drugs (such as cortisone), low-fiber diets, stress, and food allergies (especially dairy). All of these factors add to the toxic load of the body and decrease nutrient reserves. Prolonged use of antacids to treat this GI problem (and others) can adversely affect digestion and create other problems by promoting the growth of bacteria and fungus, leading to intestinal toxemia.

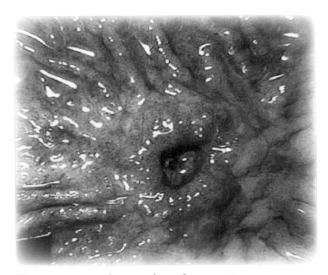

*This is an internal view of an ulcer.*

**Inflammatory Bowel Diseases**

The inflammatory bowel diseases (Crohn's disease and ulcerative colitis) are potentially serious bowel disorders involving inflammation of the bowel or GI tract, along with such symptoms as bloody diarrhea, abdominal pain, weight loss, nausea and vomiting. Ulcerative colitis affects only the surface membrane of the rectum and/or sigmoid colon, while Crohn's disease affects all

layers of the bowel wall and may encompass the entire GI tract (though usually is confined to the ileum and/or colon). While the cause of IBD is unknown, it is believed to be an autoimmune disorder. Food sensitivities and poor nutrition are thought to be major causative factors. Genetics are also thought to play a significant role. The hallmark of IBD, inflammation, is often the result of poor digestion. The putrefaction or decomposition of proteins by anaerobic microbes (those not requiring oxygen) leads to toxicity and inflammation.

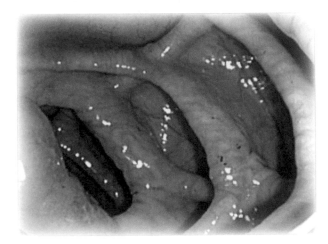

*Crohn's disease in the ileocecal valve*

**PMS and Other Female Disorders**

Liver dysfunction can give rise to premenstrual syndrome, as well as other female problems, because it adversely affects the hormonal system (as well as other critical systems). The liver is responsible for manufacturing estrogen, breaking it down and eliminating it from the body. When it is overworked and congested, it fails to adequately perform this function. Consequently, estrogen accumulates in body tissues. Estrogen build-up can lead to female problems and has been correlated with cancer. Additionally, when the liver is overloaded, toxins may be stored in the uterus (as well as other organs) to be released during menstruation.

These are just a few of the many conditions in which toxicity is a major cause or contributing factor. By keeping the channels of elimination clear, using the methods described in Chapter 6, you will do much toward eliminating those conditions that give rise to chronic disease.

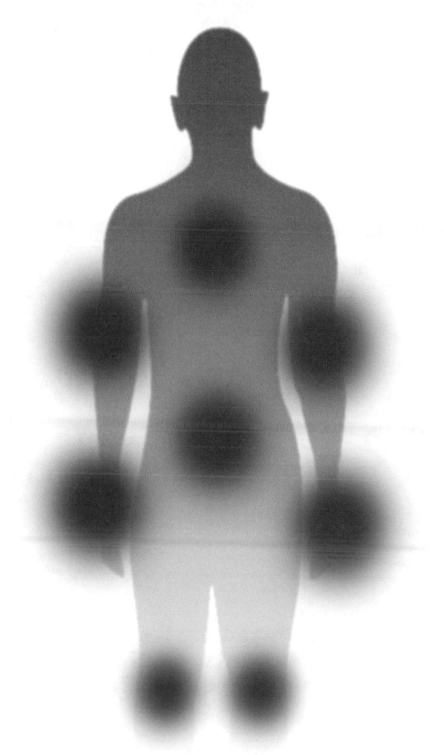

*If not eliminated properly, toxins will remain in the body, eventually settling in tissues and organs. As toxins are retained, irritation and inflammation occur resulting in chronic diseases.*

# Chapter 4: How Do I Know If I'm Toxic?

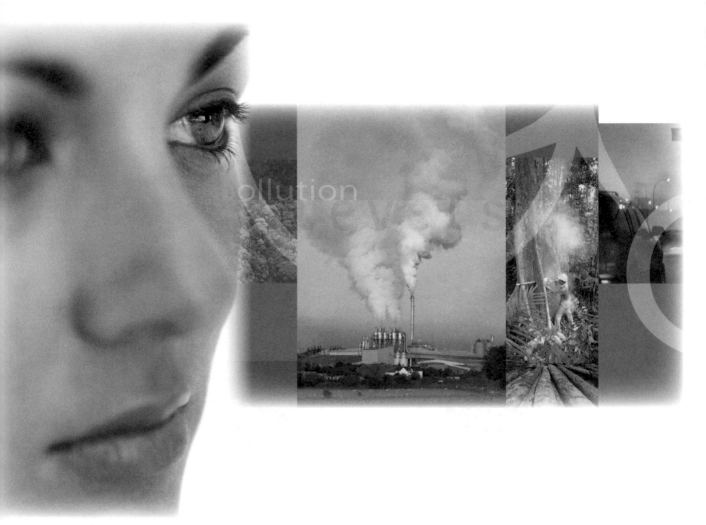

## "Everyone in the United States carries more than 100 chemical pollutants, pesticides, and toxic metals in their bodies."

*Environmental Working Group*

If you're alive on planet earth today, you're toxic to some degree — guaranteed! The question is, "How toxic are you?" The questionnaire on the next page will give you some idea.

## Read each question, and then place a one or zero on the line to the right of the question.

1. Do you brush your teeth daily?
   YES = 1  NO = 0  ___

2. Do you have 'silver' dental fillings?
   YES = 0  NO = 1  ___

3. Have you ever had tooth extractions and/or root canal fillings?
   YES = 0  NO = 1  ___

4. Do you use unfiltered tap water to brush your teeth, shower, make coffee or drink?
   YES = 0  NO = 1  ___

5. Do you have one bowel movement or more every day?
   YES = 1  NO = 0  ___

6. Do you use commercial household cleaners, cosmetics or anti-perspirants?
   YES = 0  NO = 1  ___

7. Have you ever taken prescription medications or over-the-counter medications?
   YES = 0  NO = 1  ___

8. Do you have wall-to-wall carpet in your home or office?
   YES = 0  NO = 1  ___

9. Do you prepare food in a microwave oven and/or use a cell phone?
   YES = 0  NO = 1  ___

10. Do you eat commercial (non-organic) vegetables, fruits or meat?
    YES = 0  NO = 1  ___

11. Do you wear clothes that have been dry-cleaned?
    YES = 0  NO = 1  ___

12. Do you wear synthetic materials (such as polyester)?
    YES = 0  NO = 1  ___

13. Do you eat processed food or "fast food?"
    YES = 0  NO = 1  ___

14. Have you ever smoked or been exposed to second-hand smoke?
    YES = 0  NO = 1  ___

15. Do you spend some time outdoors each day?
    YES = 1  NO = 0  ___

16. Do you eat in restaurants more than twice weekly?
    YES = 0  NO = 1  ___

17. Do you use bug spray in your home or have a pest control service?
    YES = 0  NO = 1  ___

18. Do you use weed killer on your lawn?
    YES = 0  NO = 1  ___

19. Do you dye your hair?
    YES = 0  NO = 1  ___

20. Do you use cologne or perfume?
    YES = 0  NO = 1  ___

21. Are you overweight, underweight or do you have cellulite deposits?
    YES = 0  NO = 1  ___

22. Does your occupation expose you to toxins?
    YES = 0  NO = 1  ___

23. Do you drink alcoholic beverages regularly?
    YES – 0  NO = 1  ___

24. Do you have any of the following symptoms:

    Sensitivity to perfume or other chemical odors
    YES = 0  NO = 1  ___

    Persistent joint and/or muscle pain
    YES = 0  NO = 1  ___

    Chronic infections
    YES = 0  NO = 1  ___

    Depression
    YES = 0  NO = 1  ___

    Fatigue
    YES = 0  NO = 1  ___

    Headaches
    YES = 0  NO = 1  ___

**TOTAL SCORE:** ___

---

*The lower your score, the greater the potential toxic burden you may be carrying and the more you may benefit from a detoxification program. (If you have a perfect score of 29, you are not living on planet earth in the 21st century, or you are living a very sheltered life!) Those with a very low score may need to take a slower, more gradual approach to cleansing in order to avoid possible cleansing reactions. A cleansing reaction, also known as a Herxheimer Reaction, is the temporary physical discomfort that may result if toxins are released faster than your body can get rid of them. This may result in such symptoms as fever, fatigue, diarrhea, cramps, headache, increased thirst, appetite loss, flu-like conditions, skin eruption or irritations. These reactions are generally short-lived (often just a day or two, but usually no longer than a week). Symptoms may range from mild to severe, depending upon the rate of cleansing. You'll read more about the cleansing reaction and how to bypass it in the next section.*

# Chapter 5: **Natural Solutions**

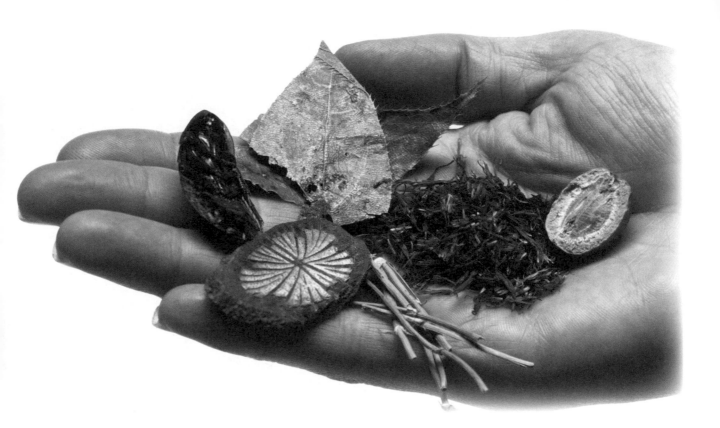

## Quantum physicists have proven through radioactive isotope studies that 98% of the atoms in your body are replaced within one year.

In three months your body produces an entirely new skeleton. Every six weeks, all the cells have been replaced in your liver. You have a new stomach lining every five days. You are continually replacing old blood cells with new ones. Your skin is sloughing off dead cells and producing a new skin monthly. The proteins in your muscles are in a constant state of flux as amino acids are catabolized and new muscle tissue is synthesized. Even your actual DNA as physical cells were not there six weeks ago.

*From Deepak Chopra's Magical Mind, Magical Body*

The human body has remarkable recuperative capacity when properly nourished, maintained and detoxified. While detoxification is a natural function of the body, as we've seen, our elimination channels can become clogged due to toxic overload and/or poor diet. To improve their functioning, we want to follow a comprehensive detoxification program. Such a practice, while unfamiliar to many, really is quite natural and beneficial. We regularly clean our homes, our cars and our outer bodies, so why neglect the inner body? We have nothing to lose but our toxins!

Many people view detoxification in a very narrow sense, seeing it as synonymous with colon cleansing. As we've learned, the colon is a major organ of elimination. When it's not working properly, toxins can be retained in the body. Therefore, colon cleansing is indeed very important. However, you'll recall that we have six other elimination channels as well. To achieve optimal cleansing results, we'll want to nourish and support all of these other channels as well as the colon. Doing this often requires pronounced changes in lifestyle and diet. Such changes will include reduction of exposure to toxins, as well as a detoxification program to eliminate toxins stored in the body. Such internal cleansing is best accomplished through appropriate use of herbal cleanses, saunas, cleansing diets or short fasts, and colon hydrotherapy (the therapeutic infusion of water into the colon for the purpose of reducing its waste content). All of these forms of cleansing have been practiced historically throughout virtually every culture in one form or another as indicated below.

# The History of Internal Cleansing

### History of Herbs

A tradition of herbal cleansing is recorded in the cultures of the ancient Sumerians, Egyptians, Romans, Greeks, Chinese, Europeans and American and Asian Indians. The Chinese have a long and rich herbal tradition, dating back some 5,000 years. They count their medicinal herbs in the thousands, as compared to the hundreds used therapeutically in Western societies. The therapeutic use of herbal preparations is also an integral part of Ayurvedic Medicine, an ancient Indian system of healing that has its roots in Vedic culture. The

American Indians also relied heavily upon the healing properties of herbs. In fact, many of the over-the-counter drugs and prescription drugs in use today in our society are derived from Native American herbs. All cultures have traditionally used eliminative herbs that have laxative, diuretic (increases urine flow), diaphoretic (sweat-inducing) and blood purifying properties to remove toxins from the body.

### History of Saunas

Saunas were developed in Finland centuries ago and have been used throughout the ages by people all over the world for their health benefits. Because of the heat they produce, saunas help your body perspire, thus promoting elimination of stored toxins through the skin, the largest major organ of elimination. Heat causes toxins to be released from cells into the lymphatic fluid. Since sweat is manufactured from lymphatic fluid, the toxins from the lymph are released when your body perspires. Releasing toxins through sweat also helps take the toxic load off the kidneys and liver, enabling them to function more efficiently, and it relaxes muscles, easing aches and pains. This "sweat therapy" is known technically as *hyperthermic* therapy.

Various forms of hyperthermic therapy have been used historically to promote elimination of toxins from the body. Native Americans have traditionally used the sweat lodge ceremony, which has existed in different forms in many other cultures, as a means of physical healing and spiritual connection. Typically, a sweat lodge is made of wooden poles that are covered with either blankets or canvas. A pit containing hot rocks is located in the center of the structure. Once participants are seated inside the lodge, the door is closed, and the ceremony takes place in darkness. It may involve a ritual consisting of prayers, chants, drumming and invocations, or it may be held in silence. Traditionally, each sweat consists of four 20- to 30-minute sessions. The sweating brought on by the steam from the hot rocks removes toxins from the body. The heat stimulates the endocrine glands. And the negative ions released into the air help alleviate tension and fatigue.[1]

Another form of hyperthermic therapy is the detoxification bath (described in subsequent pages of this section). Such baths have been long used by naturopaths and by spas in Germany.

## History of Fasting

Fasting is another time-honored cleansing tradition, one that dates back thousands of years. During a fast, no solid food is consumed, only liquids. Strict fasts allow only the ingestion of water, while more permissive ones focus on fresh juices, which are excellent sources of enzymes and antioxidant nutrients that assist in toxin removal. Some liberal "fasts" are actually monofood diets, where only a single food, usually a fruit, is consumed.

Throughout the ages, people of all faiths have fasted for religious purposes, for spiritual purification and as a means of communing with God. Others, including some doctors, have fasted, or recommended fasting, for the health benefits it confers. The "Natural Hygiene" movement (which dates back to the early 1800s) has long endorsed supervised water fasting as a means of restoring health. Juice fasting has been used extensively throughout the 20th and into the 21st century in European health clinics and elsewhere.

Fasting helps the body detoxify itself. During the fasting period, the digestive organs are put "on vacation." Digestion requires a greater output of energy than any other bodily process. During a fast, energy that would have been used to digest food is instead used to heal the body. During the fast, the body eliminates toxins that have built up in fatty tissue throughout the years, compromising health. These benefits, coupled with evidence showing that regulated fasting contributes to longer life, prompt some physicians to endorse fasting as a beneficial therapy. Others, however, warn against fasting for extended periods of time without supervision. James F. Balch, MD, and Phyllis A. Balch, CNC, list the following specific benefits of fasting[2]:

- The natural process of toxin excretion continues, while the influx of new toxins is reduced. This results in a reduction of total body toxicity.
- The energy usually used for digestion is redirected to immune function, cell growth and eliminatory processes.
- The immune system's workload is greatly reduced, and the digestive tract is spared any inflammation due to allergic reactions to food.
- Due to a lowering of serum fats that thin the blood, tissue oxygenation is increased, and white blood cells are moved more efficiently.

- Fat-stored chemicals, such as pesticides and drugs, are released.
- Physical awareness and sensitivity to diet and surroundings are increased.

There are many changes that take place in your body when you're fasting: the core temperature will decrease; blood pressure, pulse and metabolic rate will be lowered; and your breathing will slow down. Because of the powerful effect the process can have on your body, do not consider embarking on a fast without first consulting your doctor if you are pregnant or lactating, on any type of medication, or have any sort of ailment.

Some people fast to regain their health. Others fast periodically, often at the beginning of each new season as a preventive health measure. In either case, and no matter what type of fast is undertaken, it's important while fasting to limit physical activity, and rest as much as possible, though some people do feel energized as toxins leave the body.

## History of Colon Hydrotherapy

Hydrotherapy, as its name implies, is water therapy. The most simple and popular form of colon hydrotherapy is the enema. The enema involves infusion of water into the anus. This practice is referenced as far back in medical history as the first century A.D. by Galen, considered the greatest physician since Hippocrates.

Initially, enemas were the province of the medical community, though their practice was turned over to apprentices, barbers and attendants, rather than being administered directly by the physician. The use of enema syringes, which were called *clysters*, became wildly popular in the 17th century. No home was without one! The fluid carried in the clyster was often embellished with color and fragrance, and it was not uncommon for people to have as many as three to four daily rectal infusions. Monarchs were particularly privileged in this regard: history records that Louis XIII received more than 200 enemas in one single year! As time passed, "enema mania" faded, improvements were made in the process, and, by the early 19th century, colon hydrotherapy became once again the province of the medical community.

At times, medications, nutrients and other therapeutic substances have been administered via enemas. One of the most interesting of these substances has been coffee. Not only are coffee enemas referenced in the literature of folk medicine, they were even listed in the *Merck Manual* (a major reference book used by medical doctors) until 1977![3] While coffee enemas have some benefit to the colon, their major therapeutic value lies in the effect of the caffeine upon the liver and gallbladder. Among of the many benefits of coffee enemas are:

- Increased peristalsis
- Discharge of toxins from the bile duct
- Stimulation of glutathione production (which helps liver detoxification pathways)
- Breakdown of fat that has accumulated in the liver cells

The coffee enema is a form of *retention enema*, one that is held in or retained in the body for a period of time, sometimes for a matter of minutes, sometimes overnight. Retention is not difficult since typically only one to two cups of liquid is used.

Wheat grass retention enemas are sometimes used therapeutically by natural healthcare practitioners — 1 oz. of wheat grass juice to 1 cup of warm water. Wheat grass is highly beneficial as it contains all nutrients needed for healing. Retention enemas of probiotics have been effectively used to replenish beneficial bacteria in the colon.

## Coffee Enema

- Add 6 tablespoons of ground organic coffee (not decaffeinated or instant) to 2 quarts of purified or distilled water.
- Boil for 15 minutes.
- Cool to room temperature.
- Strain.
- Infuse one pint; retain for 15 minutes.
- Refrigerate the remaining coffee.

In the 1900s J.H. Kellogg, MD, of Battle Creek, Michigan (and cornflakes fame) popularized colon hydrotherapy in the US. He reported in 1917 in the *Journal of the American Medical Association* that he had successfully treated all but 20 of 40,000 gastrointestinal patients using no surgery — only diet, exercise and enemas.

Word of Dr. Kellogg's successful therapeutic use of enemas led to the development of advanced colon cleansing equipment to perform the colon-cleansing procedures known as *colonics* or *colonic irrigations*. Their practice, like that of enemas, is based on the recognition that a sluggish colon leads to re-absorption of toxins in the body.

This recognition has its roots in antiquity. Colon hydrotherapy was first recorded in ancient Egyptian documents. It was also mentioned in the writings of the Sumerians, Chinese, Hindus, Greeks and Romans. It is said that the practice of colon hydrotherapy in its most basic form, the enema, was passed down from the gods to the Egyptians. Dr. Otto Bettman describes the occasion:

"The god of medicine and science had landed on the water in the form of a sacred ibis. Filling his beak with water, he had injected it into his anus. The doctors took the hint, and the result was a great boon to humanity, the Divine Clyster".[4]

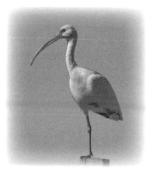

By the 1950s, colon hydrotherapy was flourishing in the United States. In fact, prestigious Beverly Boulevard in Los Angeles, California was then known as "colonic row." By the mid-1960s, however, the use of colon hydrotherapy had slowly dwindled. By the early 1970s, most colon hydrotherapy instruments were removed from hospitals and nursing homes, being displaced by the use of prescription laxatives and surgery. At this point in time, the use of colon hydrotherapy left the domain of medicine, becoming once again the domain of the lay practitioner.

The late Dr. Bernard Jensen, DC, among many other contributions to the natural health field, popularized the use of colon hydrotherapy in conjunction with herbs in his classic book, *Tissue Cleansing Through Bowel Management*, introduced in 1981. In this book, Dr. Jensen detailed an intensive seven-day cleansing program pioneered by the late Dr. V.E. Irons. The program features the use of cleansing drinks containing fiber and clay water (which absorbs toxins), specific supplements designed to nourish the body and loosen accumulations on the bowel wall, and twice-daily *colemas* (colon therapy with a colon-cleansing device that uses the force of gravity to infuse large amounts of water into the colon). The supplements and drinks specified in the program substitute for solid food for the seven-day period. Dr. Jensen's book contains some very graphic and impressive photographs showing both the morbid matter that can build up in the colon and the spectacular healing (of the skin) that can occur as a result of removing it.

## Colon Hydrotherapy Today

A colonic is basically an extended and more complete form of enema. Both the enema and the colonic involve the infusion of water into the colon through the anal opening. However, the enema is a one-time infusion of water into the rectum. The patient takes in as much as a quart of water, holds it for a time, and then releases it directly into the toilet. In contrast, colonic treatments (now known as colon hydrotherapy sessions) involve repeated infusions of filtered, warm water into all segments of the colon by a certified colon therapist. During the course of a treatment, the patient lies comfortably on his or her back.

Colon hydrotherapists are trained to use massage techniques to help relax abdominal muscles and ensure that all areas of the colon are adequately irrigated. While the colon is filled and emptied a few times during one 45-minute session, there is no need for the client to leave the table to expel the water. The passage of the water in and out of the colon is controlled by the therapist who operates the colonic apparatus, while the client lies still on the table. As the water leaves the body, it passes through a clear viewing tube, allowing both client and therapist to see what is being eliminated from the colon. In addition to fecal matter, gas bubbles, mucus and parasites are often seen.

# Conditions That May Benefit from Colon Hydrotherapy

Acne
Allergies
Arthritis
Asthma
Attention Deficit Disorder
Body odor
Brittle nails
Brittle hair
Chest pain
Chronic fatigue
Cold hands and feet
Colitis
Constipation
Fibromyalgia
Headaches
Hypertension
Irritable Bowel Syndrome
Joint aches
Memory lapses
Mouth sores
Multiple sclerosis
Muscle pain
Nausea
Peptic ulcer
Peripheral neuropathies
Pigmentation
Poor posture
Potbelly
Seizures
Skin rashes
Spastic colon
Toxic environmental exposure

Chart 1

There is no odor or health risk involved in the colonic procedure when performed properly by a trained, certified colon therapist. Therapeutic benefits of colon hydrotherapy include improved tone of colonic muscles, reduced stagnation of intestinal contents, reduced toxic waste absorption and the thorough cleansing and balancing of the colon.

Your colon can hold a great deal of waste material. That which is not eliminated promptly putrefies, adding to the toxic load of your body. Many people with "potbellies" may actually have several pounds of old, hardened fecal matter lodged within their colons. While colon hydrotherapy is not actually a weight loss procedure, it does often result in significant weight loss due to its ability to efficiently reduce the toxic burden of the large intestine. Furthermore, several ailments have been associated with colon toxicity. People with conditions listed in Chart 1 may benefit from colon hydrotherapy.

Colon hydrotherapy has helped many people overcome constipation. Unlike chemical laxatives, it does not encourage dependency, but rather helps to tone the bowel, gently prompting it to resume normal functioning.

Your cleansing, as well as overall health, will be aided significantly by the addition of colon hydrotherapy sessions. Such therapy stimulates the liver, your body's major organ of detoxification, helping it to eliminate toxins.

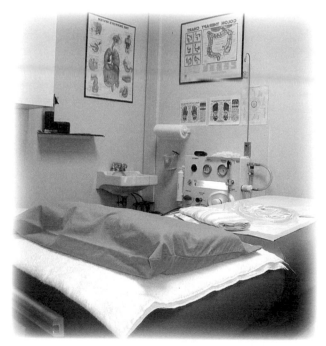

*This is a photo of a typical colon therapy room.*

Colon hydrotherapy also benefits your body's lymphatic system, for when the intestinal walls are impacted, the lymphatic system retains and continuously re-circulates cellular waste. Your lymphatic system (your body's sewage system) become stagnant when the normally clear lymph fluid becomes thick with cellular debris, toxins, microorganisms and dietary fats. Thickened, stagnant lymph contributes to fatigue, malaise (vague feeling of illness) and weight gain, especially around the abdomen, hips and buttocks.[5]

Look for a colon therapist certified by the International Association for Colon Hydrotherapy (I-ACT). These therapists use FDA-registered equipment, disposable rectal nozzles (called speculums) and filtered water. I-ACT is the worldwide certifying body for colon hydrotherapists. The organization works in conjunction with local municipalities to regulate colon hydrotherapy by establishing standards and guidelines.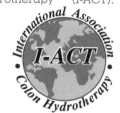

If you are able to add one or more colon hydrotherapy sessions to your cleansing regime, it can greatly facilitate your progress, and help to prevent or alleviate the symptoms associated with cleansing reations (and with colon toxicity). Your colon therapist, following your initial session, can give guidelines about suggested frequency and duration of treatment. If colon hydrotherapy is not an option for you, enemas may be used instead. Though not as thorough as colonics, they do facilitate colon cleansing.

You can enhance your colon cleansing efforts if you simulate the natural squatting posture when you sit on the toilet to have a bowel movement. This can be done easily by elevating your feet while seated on the commode, resting them on a special platform called a Life Step™.

## Fasting Today

Foods such as fatty meats, white flour, sugar and dairy products can clog the channels of elimination. There are also foods that **build** (make us stronger and more resilient), those that **cleanse** (relieve the toxic burden) and those that both **cleanse and build**. Proteins, such as meat and eggs, are the major builders. Most fruits

# Detoxification Diet

- **Eat plenty of lean meats** (flank steak, top sirloin steak, London broil ) plus chicken and turkey breasts, wild game, and fish. Choose the meat of organically raised, pastured animals (those that eat grass, not grains) whenever possible. Choose smaller fish such as flounder, sole, pollock and halibut over the large ones like swordfish, shark and tuna, which tend to accumulate more mercury. Avoid raw fish (can be a source of parasites). Choose wild fish, including salmon, over farm-raised fish, whose diet is often lacking in omega-3 fatty acids.
- **Avoid fatty meats.** Bacon, beef ribs, chicken and turkey legs, thighs, wings and skin, fatty beef roasts, fatty cuts of beef, fatty ground beef, fatty pork chops, fatty pork roasts, lamb chops, lamb roasts, leg of lamb, pork ribs, pork sausage and T-bone steaks.
- **Avoid or minimize salted foods.** Deli meats, hot dogs, smoked, dried and salted fish and meat, bacon, cheese, ham, most commercial salad dressings and condiments, pickled foods, pork rinds, processed meats, salted nuts, salted spices, sausages and olives.
- **Eggs are permitted.** Limit to six per week, and choose free-range organic.
- **Avoid or minimize use of table salt.** Use unprocessed sea salt sparingly.
- **Eliminate sugars and artificial sweeteners, as well as foods containing them.** This includes sucrose (or table sugar), lactose (milk sugar found in dairy products), honey, fructose (fruit sugar), molasses, maple syrup and other concentrated sweeteners. A moderate amount of the herbs stevia or lo han may be used as a sweetener when needed. All sodas, diet and regular, are to be strictly avoided.
- **Limit grains.** Choose those that do not contain gluten (such as corn, millet, teff and quinoa). Only whole grains are recommended, used sparingly — no more than four servings daily (one-half to one cup = one serving). Avoid wheat bread and wheat-based products; try sprouted grain ("Ezekiel") bread or millet bread. Avoid all processed foods made with refined cereal grains — commercial rolls, pasta, noodles, muffins, waffles, cookies, cake, doughnuts, pancakes and crackers.
- **Eat fruits freely.** (if candida is not a problem), favoring those that have a low glycemic index (a measurement of how quickly the body breaks down carbohydrates into glucose in the bloodstream). These would include berries of all sorts, pears, peaches, plums, dried apricots, cherries, bananas, apples, grapefruit, oranges, kiwis and grapes.
- **Eat non-starchy vegetables freely.** Minimize intake of starchy vegetables (starchy tubers, cassava root, manioc, potatoes of all types, tapioca pudding and yams) and legumes (all beans, peas and lentils).
- **Avoid all canned, bottled and frozen juices.** As well as freshly prepared fruit juices (which lack the fiber of fresh fruit and have a much higher glycemic index). Stick with freshly prepared vegetable juices. Emphasize the green juices.
- **Avoid commercial dairy products.** Milk, sour cream, buttermilk, cheeses, margarine and other milk products. The exceptions are butter and plain (not low-fat or no-fat) yogurt, in small amounts — no more than one-half a cup per day.
- **Avoid white potatoes, russets, yams and sweet potatoes.** A moderate amount of red potatoes is permitted.
- **Avoid or greatly minimize intake of alcoholic beverages.**
- **Avoid or limit coffee and tea.** Choose organic, decaffeinated coffee and/or herbal teas instead.
- **Eat nuts and seeds in moderation.** Always soak them in water overnight before eating to deactivate enzyme inhibitors.

The above guidelines represent a modified Paleolithic Diet, which features lean meat, fresh fruit and vegetables. Such an eating plan is based on the premise that we were designed to thrive on the foods that our ancient ancestors ate, the hunter-gatherer diet that preceded the age of agriculture. Consuming an abundance of lean meat provides plenty of protein to lower cholesterol, improve insulin sensitivity, speed up metabolism, satisfy appetite and aid in weight loss.

Chart 2

are aggressive cleansers, while vegetables have both a cleansing and building effect on the body. Ideally, a detoxification diet will feature cleansing foods, but contain enough of the building ones to prevent undue discomfort brought on by too rapid release of toxins. An extreme cleansing or detoxification program such as a water fast (where no food at all is eaten and no beverage consumed other than water), fruit diet or prolonged juice "fast" is not recommended. While such practices do cleanse and accomplish the purpose of giving the digestive organs a rest so that energy may be diverted to healing, they may also bring on a powerful cleansing reaction (Herxheimer reaction) when toxins are released faster than they can be eliminated, causing a great deal of discomfort. A total fast can be debilitating for those with little or no nutritional reserves. A fruit diet, while accomplishing the task of cleansing, may also cause problems by eliciting a strong insulin response, thereby leading to blood sugar imbalances and other problems associated with carbohydrate over-consumption.

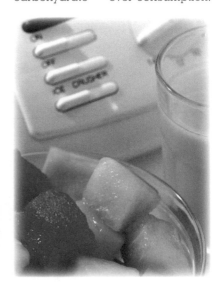

Most fruits, due to their high sugar content, also provide nourishment for any fungal organisms we may be harboring, and can give rise to candida overgrowth and such attendant problems as fatigue, allergies, digestive problems and brain fog.

A short fast of three days' duration, featuring freshly prepared vegetable juices (especially green juices), can be most beneficial to the body and is an excellent way to jump-start your cleansing program, for fresh juices are nutrient-dense, and their nutrients are readily available for the body to use. Eat a light meal for supper the evening before you begin your juice fast. Try combining leafy greens like spinach with a juicy green like cucumber in a base of carrot juice. The addition of garlic or fresh ginger will enhance the therapeutic value (and taste) of your creation. Make fresh juices from a recipe book or experiment with creating your own recipes. Be sure to drink your juice immediately after preparing it, as it will not store well. Start slowly, drinking just a few ounces, or dilute the juice with water until you become accustomed to the taste. Prepare fresh juice as often as possible throughout the day. Drink water when not drinking vegetable juice, striving to consume one-half ounce for every pound of body weight throughout the day (100-pound person drinks 50 ounces per day). Herbal tea is also permissible, but avoid coffee, sodas, fruit juice and pre-packaged juices of any kind while on a juice fast. At the end of your three-day juice fast, introduce solid foods gradually, starting with the lighter ones like non-starchy vegetables or citrus fruit. By dinner of the first day following a fast, you may add back starches, but wait another day before adding heavy protein foods like meat.

To cleanse effectively but safely, follow your three-day fast with a balanced diet of cleansing and building foods, as well as elimination of all processed foods. The specifics of such a detoxification diet are outlined in chart 2.

Olive oil and/or coconut oil are suggested for use with cooking. Olive oil is also useful as (or in) a salad dressing. Unrefined extra virgin olive oil is the best choice. Flax oil is also good in a salad dressing.

Adhering to a diet such as this, along with the use of appropriate herbal supplements to strengthen and support your body's detoxification channels, can do much to lessen the toxic load of your body. Such a cleanse is recommended on at least an annual basis,

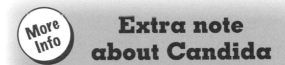

# Extra note about Candida

If you have been diagnosed with *Candida albicans* or suspect you may have a fungal problem, you will additionally want to do the following:

- Avoid peanuts and peanut butter. These have a high content of aflatoxins, a carcinogenic mold. Almond butter, cashew butter, tahini (sesame seed butter) or other nut or seed butters may be substituted. These should be refrigerated to avoid rancidity.
- Avoid mushrooms and all types of cheeses. These either contain, or actually are, molds or yeasts.
- Avoid beer, wine and other alcoholic beverages (all yeast-containing), as well as commercial sauerkraut, commercial salad dressings, all types of vinegars, soy sauce, Worcestershire sauce, horseradish, pickles, relish, green olives, commercial soups, potato chips and dry roasted nuts.
- Avoid or limit coffee, coffee substitutes, tea, pepper, many spices and tobacco. These foods tend to acquire molds or yeast in the drying process. Even herb teas may become moldy, so their use should be limited, especially for sensitive individuals. Teas with anti-fungal properties include pau d'arco, chamomile, bergamot, hyssop, alfalfa, angelica root and lemon grass. Pau d'arco, in particular, has been shown to be effective in killing candida. If you must have your coffee, limit yourself to two cups per day of organic decaffeinated (that has been decaffeinated using a chemical-free water process).

but may be done more often. Some people like to embark upon a cleansing program at the beginning of every new season. Such regimens can be enhanced through addition of colon hydrotherapy and the use of saunas and/or soaks, all of which gently accelerate the release of toxins without causing excessive stress to the body. These topics are discussed below. Exercise, gentle or vigorous, depending upon your individual condition, is vital during this period of time to stimulate circulation, facilitating the release of toxins.

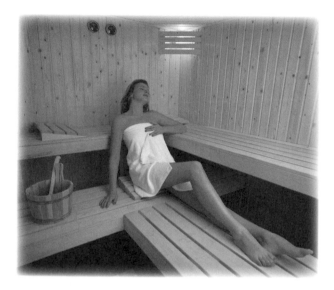

## Saunas, Soaks and Skin Brushing

Sweating occurs naturally during activity such as strenuous exercise, exposure to the sun or being in a warm room. Saunas (dry heat), steam baths (wet heat) and even tub baths can create sweat intentionally for therapeutic purposes.

Raising the core temperature of your body through the hyperthermic effect has been shown to have a favorable impact upon the immune system. It is one of the few known ways to stimulate increased production of growth hormone, which helps your body shed fat, while maintaining lean muscle mass. Hyperthermic therapy also helps to restore autonomic nervous system function. This system governs muscle tension, sweating, blood pressure, digestion and balance. The autonomic nervous system is often dysfunctional in people with chronic fatigue and fibromyalgia (a chronic disease involving pain in muscles and joints).

For this reason, people with these conditions can gain particular benefit from sauna therapy, of which there are two types: conventional sauna and infrared sauna.

A conventional sauna heats the air either electrically or by the burning of wood. Your skin perspires as a result of direct contact with the hot air. Typically, temperatures of 180 to 235 degrees Fahrenheit are used to induce sweating. These high temperatures increase cardiac load in the same way that aerobic exercise does.

Hal Huggins, DDS, an authority on mercury detoxification, recommends use of the sauna for detoxification. He suggests that the ill or sensitive patient start out at a temperature of 135 degrees, work up to staying in the sauna for 45 minutes without discomfort and leave the sauna at any sign of discomfort. Once 135 degrees is comfortably tolerated for 45 minutes, temperature may be gradually increased to 145 degrees.[6] (These temperatures apply to a conventional sauna, not infrared.)

In recent years, infrared saunas have been widely used for their superior therapeutic effect. Infrared heat is radiant heat. It heats objects directly without heating the air in between. In the infrared sauna, only 20% of the infrared energy heats the air; the other 80% is directly converted to heat within the body. The result is that your body perspires more quickly at lower temperatures than in a conventional sauna. The heat also penetrates more deeply, although without the discomfort and draining effect often experienced in a conventionally heated sauna. An infrared sauna produces two to three times more sweat volume, and because of the lower temperatures used (110-130 degrees), it is considered safer for those at cardiovascular risk.

People suffering from sports injuries, arthritis, chronic fatigue and fibromyalgia, as well as other painful conditions, have benefited from the use of infrared saunas. These saunas accelerate the removal of toxic metals, as well as organic toxins like PCBs and pesticide residues — chemicals that are stored in the fatty tissues of the body and are not easily dislodged. The heat produced in infrared saunas is extremely beneficial for those suffering from such skin conditions as acne, eczema and psoriasis. The sweating caused by deep heat helps eliminate dead skin cells, reduces cellulite deposits and improves skin tone and elasticity. Weight loss is facilitated through use of an infrared sauna, in part due to the increase in growth hormone that it produces. It has been calculated that one can burn 600 calories in 30 minutes in an infrared sauna. Health benefits can certainly be obtained in a conventional sauna or steam bath as well, but the infrared sauna has a greater range of therapeutic efficiency, especially for detoxification. The infrared sauna actually has an energizing effect on users, making them feel good as toxins are eliminated.

According to detoxification expert, Sherry A. Rogers, MD, "A sauna program is the only known way of getting rid of twentieth century man-made chemicals"[7] such as PCBs, dioxins, pesticides and phthalates (plasticizers). As Dr. Rogers points out, saunas have helped detoxify people who have had significant toxic exposure: drug addicts, fire fighters, Vietnam veterans (exposed to Agent Orange), farmers, and pesticide pilots, to name a few. Saunas are also an excellent detoxification aid for people with multiple chemical sensitivities and others with "incurable" symptoms.

Conventional saunas and steam baths are generally found in gymnasiums and health spas. Infrared saunas are more apt to be found in clinics run by holistic practitioners. People with health problems should consult a natural healthcare practitioner before using either type of sauna.

If you don't have access to a sauna or steam bath, you may want to do your own detoxification bath at home. This is prepared by filling a clean tub with hot filtered water (a shower filter or whole house filter is recommended). Make the water as hot as you can comfortably tolerate. There are a number of therapeutic substances that may be used in the bath water. One is Epsom salts, which contains magnesium (which relaxes muscles) and sulfur (which aids in detoxification and helps increase blood supply to the skin). A quarter cup of Epsom salts is a good start, with a gradual increase to as much as two to four pounds per bath. Another option is ginger root. Ginger helps the body to sweat, so toxins are drawn to the skin's surface. To prepare the ginger bath, place half-inch slices of fresh ginger in boiling water; then turn off the heat, and steep for 30 minutes. Remove the ginger, and pour the water into the tub.[8]

 **Detox Bath**

Dr. Huggins suggests the following procedure for a detoxification bath:

- Bring the bath water to a temperature of 104 degrees Fahrenheit.
- Soak a bath sheet (3' x 6' towel) in the bath water.
- Get in the tub, and pull the bath sheet over you like you would a bed sheet.
- Keep the towel warm by periodically soaking it in the water.
- Leave the tub when you start to feel woozy.
- Stay in no longer than 20 minutes.
- Rinse with fresh water.
- Repeat the procedure 2–3 times per week.

Dr. Huggins states that a soak of only two to three minutes will actually produce results, while benefits are maximized at 20 minutes. Often toxic metals leave the body and are visible after the bath in the form of a powder that adheres to the tub walls. Dr. Huggins suggests that adding a cup of baking soda to the bath water will enhance the effect of the soak. After the third bath, decrease baking soda to one-half a cup, but also add one-half a cup of Epsom salts. After another three baths, add one full cup of each.[9] Other detox bath additives may include:

**Apple cider vinegar** — increases blood supply to skin, changes its pH
**Hydrogen peroxide** — used in warm water (not hot), increases oxygen at the cellular level
**Clay** — has drawing properties and alkalizing action
**Oatstraw** — good for skin conditions
**Burdock Root** — helps the body excrete uric acid; useful when rashes are present

After any type of hyperthermic therapy (and during, if possible), be sure to drink lots of water to replace fluid lost through perspiration.

In addition to detoxification through saunas and soaks, toxins may be eliminated from the skin by brushing it with a special natural bristle skin brush. This may be purchased in a health food store. Brush the skin before showering or bathing, stroking toward the heart, gently but vigorously. This will help open the pores of your skin, increase circulation and remove dead skin cells. Remember: The skin is a major organ of elimination, and brushing it regularly helps it do its job.

If you have access to some form of sauna, a steam bath or even a bathtub, you may wish to use it regularly in the manners described above to facilitate detoxification. If you are unable to do any form of heat therapy, you still can benefit from adding regular skin brushing to your daily regimen.

## Exercise

There are many forms of exercise, each offering a unique set of benefits. Generally speaking, the benefits of exercise include:[10]

- Increased stamina and energy
- Increased flexibility
- Increased blood circulation
- Increased lymphatic circulation (which aids in detoxification and increases immunity)
- Better sleep/decreased need for sleep
- Stress reduction
- Development of self-discipline
- Increased self-esteem
- Increased oxygen supply to cells and tissues
- Increased muscle strength/tone and endurance
- Release of brain chemicals called endorphins, which act as a natural tranquilizer
- Increased progesterone and decreased estrogen production in women, potentially easing PMS and cramps
- Decrease in food cravings
- Decreased blood sugar levels (which increases effectiveness of insulin)
- Weight redistribution and maintenance

Aerobic exercise takes energy from the cells, and by doing so, helps them to increase the number and size of the mitochondria (power generators) and operate more efficiently.[11] As your mitochondria increase, so too does your energy, and your ability to burn fat. Aerobic exercises include:

- Walking
- Running/jogging
- Bicycling
- Rowing
- Skiing
- Fast dancing
- Jumping rope
- Skating

If engaged in any of the above activities, you must sustain motion for at least 15 to 20 minutes in order to obtain the aerobic effect. If exercise has not been part of your daily regimen, start with a shorter period, say five minutes, and add another five-minute increment every week or so.

One of the greatest benefits of exercise is body purification, the cleansing of the blood and all body tissues.

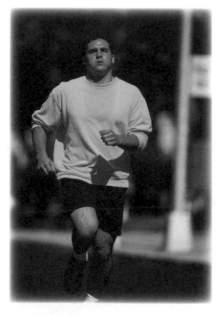

While your choice of exercise is an individual matter and should reflect your personal preferences, regular walking and/or use of a rebounder or mini-trampoline (which can incorporate a jogging or jumping motion) are encouraged here because of their simplicity, accessibility and proven benefits. Both are excellent ways of stimulating both blood and lymphatic circulation, helping to move toxins out of their storage sites and out of your body.

The simple act of walking pumps lymph nodes, concentrated in the neck, underarms, groin and behind the knees, helping to move toxins out of the body. Slow movement exercises, like yoga and tai chi, will also work the lymph glands, helping to detoxify your body, as well as stabilize structure.

If you are transitioning from a sedentary lifestyle into one that incorporates regular exercise, start slowly, with a short walk and/or a short session on the rebounder, gradually increasing the time engaged in the activity and the intensity of your effort. If walking, work up to a sustained fast pace for 15 to 20 minutes. Breathe deeply as you walk, letting arms swing in a "cross-crawl" motion, so that the right arm is swinging forward at the same time the left foot is put forward — a brisk marching movement.

Jogging on a rebounder is easier on your body than jogging on a hard surface, for as your feet hit the running surface, there is no resistance: your body is propelled upward, and you don't lose energy on the down bounce. With rebounding, there is no risk of injury to your joints.

If you're new to the rebounder, you may want to start out with a "soft walk," where you simply shift your weight from one foot to another, lifting your heels as you do so. Even this gentle motion is enough to stimulate lymph flow, helping your body to dissolve and eliminate toxins and strengthen your immune system. Rebounding so effectively moves lymphatic fluid that it has been referred to as "lymphasizing." In addition to clearing the lymph glands, rebounding will provide aerobic exercise (once you've worked up to a sustained motion for 15 to 20 minutes), oxygenating your body.

When you jump up and down on a rebounder, the force of gravity alternately pulls and then releases each cell, stimulating cellular fluid flow so that toxic material is flushed out, and nutrients are absorbed. In addition, the valves in your lymphatic system open and shut when you rebound, pumping lymphatic fluid throughout your body. During this process, not only are toxins removed, but white blood cells are also produced. Even a short (two- to three-minute) rebounding session will dramatically increase your white blood cell production, which has the net effect of increasing immunity. In addition to providing cellular cleansing and enhanced immunity, rebounding exercises the musculo-skeletal system, protects and strengthens the cardiovascular and peripheral vascular systems and helps restore bone density. It is a safe and easy-to-perform exercise for people of any age and in any physical condition. Use your rebounder at least once daily. Short, frequent rebounding sessions can be as beneficial as a single long one.

Start slowly, and don't overdo it. You may wish to start with one five-minute rebounder session per day and/or one ten-minute walk daily (or five or six times per week). You would then gradually increase your rebounding or walking time until it is doubled and/or add an extra short rebounder session, as time in your schedule permits. Another option would be to rebound and walk on alternate days. If you have another form of exercise that you prefer, by all means continue doing it. Just consider adding a little rebounding to the mix. The particulars of your program are not nearly as important as your commitment to setting up a routine and goals and sticking with them.

## The Do's and Don'ts of a Cleansing Lifestyle

The subjects discussed thus far — a detoxification diet, saunas, soaks, skin brushing, colon hydrotherapy, exercise — are all part of what we might call a "cleansing lifestyle." At the crux of your cleansing program will be specific herbal cleanses designed to assist your body in getting rid of toxins. Before discussing the specifics of the recommended herbal cleanses, let's look at some of the specific components of a healthy lifestyle. Many of the items listed below have already been discussed or mentioned in earlier sections. Strive to incorporate as many of the following recommendations as possible into your daily regimen:

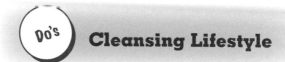

- Drink plenty of water every day (half your body's weight in ounces). Without sufficient water, toxins are reabsorbed.

- Consider investing in a good-quality water purification unit, such as a reverse osmosis system. In addition to purifying drinking water, use a shower filter or whole house filter to avoid toxic exposure from bathing and showering. Change all filters in a timely manner as per manufacturer's directions.

- Add minerals back to your water if you drink distilled or reverse osmosis water.
- Choose organic food products whenever possible.
- Invest in a good-quality air purifier — and change the filters regularly.
- Change/clean the filter in your air conditioning unit/s often.
- Use plants (spider plant, aloe, chrysanthemum, philodendron, Gerber daisies) to help filter toxins from and add oxygen to your indoor air.
- Eat plenty of fresh vegetables (preferably organically grown) daily and their juices. Fresh vegetable juices are quickly and easily absorbed, within 30 minutes of ingestion.
- Use unrefined oils. Choose coconut, sesame, flax or olive oil (preferably organic). Never cook with flax oil; it is very heat-sensitive.
- Exercise regularly. (Remember: The rebounder is great for stimulating lymphatic circulation).
- Eat plenty of raw foods. Increase the amount slowly, working your way up to 50% or more of your diet.
- Get some natural sunlight per day (about 10-15 minutes). Take off your glasses or sunglasses so that beneficial rays will not be blocked.
- Substitute all-natural (preferably organic) personal care and household products for commercial ones, which contain toxic ingredients.
- Read labels!
- Combine foods properly (especially if you suffer from digestive disturbances).
- Eat slowly, and chew your food well.

- Aluminum, stainless steel and non-stick cookware. Use porcelain or glass instead.
- Exposure to radiations from microwave ovens and cell phones. There is evidence that these can be damaging to the body.
- Artificial sweeteners. Choose stevia or lo-han instead.
- Caffeine-containing coffee and tea. Choose organic. Consider using coffee that has been decaffeinated by a chemical-free water process and/or naturally caffeine-free herbal teas.
- Synthetic fragrances. Choose essential oils instead. (Essential oils are compounds found within aromatic plants.)
- Anti-bacterial soaps. They will kill the good bacteria, along with the bad, and contribute to development of antibiotic-resistant strains of bacteria.
- Anti-perspirants. Instead use a deodorant that does not contain aluminum.
- Toxic pesticides. Choose natural products like boric acid, or find a natural pest control service.
- Drinking large amounts of liquid with your meals or immediately afterward. This can interfere with digestion.
- Wearing tight bras. They restrict lymph drainage in the chest area and under the arms.
- Overeating. This can cause digestive distress and even reduce lifespan.
- Eating when you are under stress. This is another factor that will cause digestive problems.
- Synthetic carpets. Choose natural fibers like wool, hemp, cotton or jute — manufactured without additives — or use tile instead.

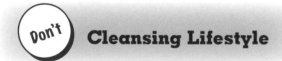

## Don't Cleansing Lifestyle

As far as possible, you'll want to avoid the following:

- Tap water. Do not use at home or away from home. Carry your own purified water with you. Store in glass, rather than plastic.
- Sodas (including diet sodas) and other junk food.
- Processed foods (refined grain products made from white sugar and flour, refined and hydrogenated oils). Minimize consumption of such products by eating out as seldom as possible and making wise food choices when you do.

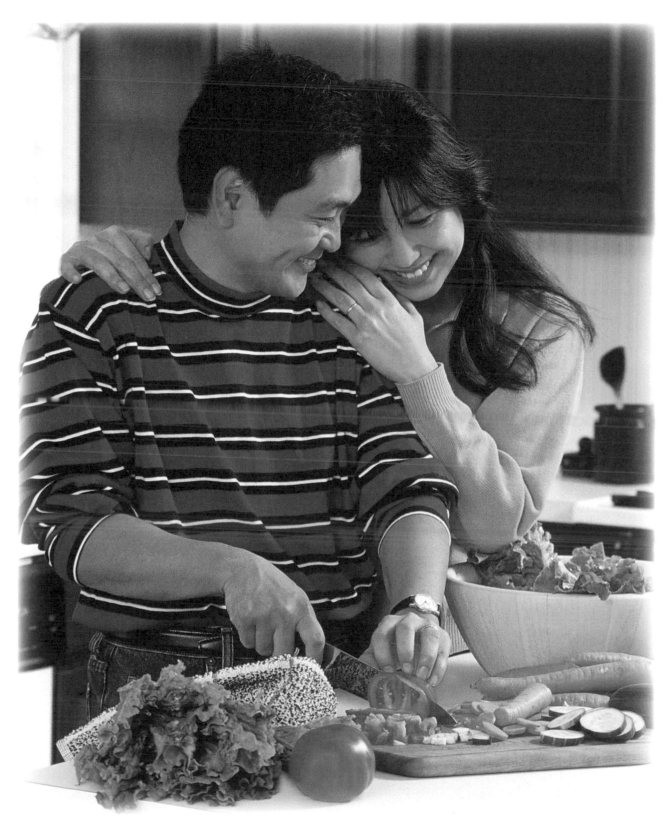

# Chapter 6: **Your Cleansing Program**

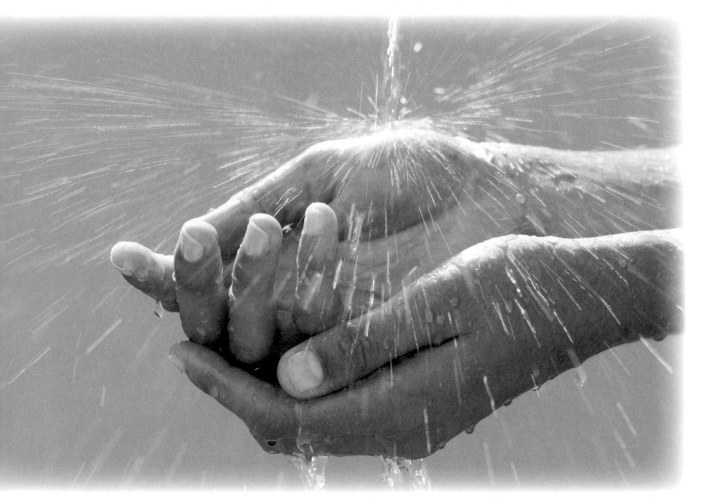

## While drugs add to the toxic burden of the body, specific herbs can actually assist the body's natural detoxification process.

The heart of your herbal detox regimen is supplementation with herbs that will help all seven of your body's elimination channels (liver, lungs, colon, kidneys, blood, skin and lymph) by means of several different mechanisms. Stimulating these channels naturally enhances the physical process of detoxification so that your body is able to rid itself of toxins without obstruction. Some of the mechanisms by which the recommended herbs enhance the detoxification process include:

- Stimulation of bile production in the liver
- Stimulation of peristalsis
- Stimulation of urine output (a diuretic effect)
- Hydration of the colon
- Stimulation of blood and lymphatic circulation
- Provision of nutritional support to strengthen organs and protect them from toxic damage
- Promotion of mucus discharge from lungs (an expectorant effect)
- Eradication of pathogens (such as fungi, viruses and bacteria)
- Prevention of fat deposits in the liver

Numerous herbs working together synergistically provide the above effects, one of the most important of which is stimulation of bile production and flow. Bile is "the yellowish brown or green fluid secreted by the liver and discharged into the duodenum (upper part of the small intestine) where it aids in the emulsification of fats, increases peristalsis and retards putrefaction."[1] Bile contains many spent body substances, including salts, acids, cholesterol, mucus, fat, dead red blood cells, toxins and other cellular debris. The liver dumps these toxic materials into the bile, which carries them into the colon so they may be flushed from the body. If bile flow is stagnant due to liver congestion, then the colon will not eliminate efficiently, and toxins will be retained. As they build up, your body will produce extra fat and extra water in an attempt to dilute toxins. The liver then becomes a key organ of elimination for the dual purposes of detoxification and weight loss. Liver support, therefore, is of central importance in any cleansing program.

While drugs add to the toxic burden of the body, specific herbs actually can assist the body's natural detoxification process. Traditionally, detoxification and cleansing are accomplished naturally through the use of eliminative herbs that act as laxatives, diuretics, diaphoretics (to produce sweating) and blood purifiers. Other herbs support the cleansing process by toning specific organs and allowing the body to heal itself.

To simplify the herbal cleansing process and maximize its effects, a four-step herbal cleansing program, which combines herbs that cleanse with those that build, is recommended. The first of these cleanses would focus on ridding the colon of accumulated toxins, while the

## Four simple steps to the herbal cleansing program

1. Focused Colon Cleanse

2. Whole Body Basic Cleanse (a two-part formula recommended)

3. Whole Body Advanced Cleanse (a two-part formula recommended)

4. Whole Body Maintenance Cleanse (a single herbal blend recommended)

last three would contain herbs that nourish and support all seven channels of elimination, making them Whole Body Cleanses. The four simple steps to the herbal cleansing program are:

1. Focused Colon Cleanse
2. Whole Body Basic Cleanse (a two-part formula recommended)
3. Whole Body Advanced Cleanse (a two-part formula recommended)
4. Whole Body Maintenance Cleanse (a single herbal blend recommended)

Upon completion of the Whole Body Cleanses, you are ready to move on to two more Focused Cleanses. These are cleanses that target specific organs or processes. These two Focused Cleanses would contain herbal combinations designed to cleanse the body tissues more deeply. The first Focused Cleanse is aimed at providing optimal support for the liver. The other is focused on reducing the body's burden of heavy metals. The desired herbal composition of the recommended six cleanses will be discussed in the sections that follow.

# Focused Colon Cleanse

Your first order of business will be to focus on colon cleansing with herbs, using a bowel cleansing formula that contains organic herbs. We want the colon to be working properly before we start to release stored toxins; otherwise, those toxins will be dumped into a clogged colon and re-circulated rather than eliminated.

Look for a bowel-cleansing formula that comes in bulk form, rather than one that is encapsulated. Ideally it would contain the organic ingredients listed in chart 1.

You'll want to take one scoop of this herbal formula one to three times per day as needed. Mix it with a tall glass of water, take separate from meals, and do not take at the same time that medication is taken. Start with the lower dose (one scoop once a day); if it doesn't produce the desired results, add a second scoop several hours later (again mixing with a tall glass of water). If you're still not getting results, take a third scoop several hours later (always with water). Your goal is to have two to three good bowel movements daily, ideally after each meal. A good bowel movement is one that is walnut brown in color, with a consistency similar to toothpaste, about the length of a banana. The stool would be free of odor, leave the body easily, settle in the toilet water and gently submerge.

While you're doing this herbal cleanse, you will also want to be following a cleansing diet and take saunas or soaks and colonics (chapter 5) whenever possible. If you are doing all of this, plus your herbal cleanse, you'll have a busy day. Since you'll have a lot to remember, you may want to create a cleansing schedule to help you stay on track with your cleansing regimen. You will have a lot of leeway as to when you do what, but as a general guideline, refer to the sample schedule provided. This schedule incorporates other nutritional supplements that will enhance the cleansing process: **H**igh Fiber, Essential **O**ils, **P**robiotics and **E**nzymes (the **H.O.P.E.** formula). Continue the Focused Colon Cleanse until the bowel is unclogged and functioning as described above.

## RECOMMENDED Focused Colon Cleanse Ingredients

- Flax Seed
- Oat Fiber
- Acacia Gum
- Fructooligosaccharides (FOS)
- Cinnamon
- Rhubarb Root
- Marshmallow
- Slippery Elm
- Okra
- Ginger Root
- Fennel
- Papaya
- Cayenne
- Coriander
- Cumin
- Gentian
- Black Pepper
- Peppermint
- Spearmint
- Cellulase

Chart 1

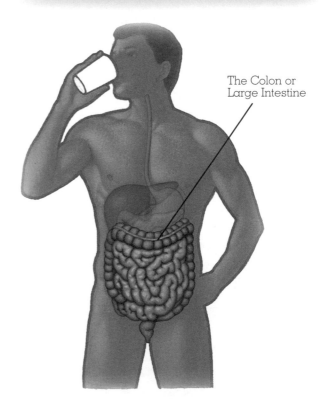

The Colon or Large Intestine

# SAMPLE
## Cleansing Schedule
(sample only, details may vary, according to your needs and schedule)

**6 AM**     Wake up. Take probiotic with a tall glass of water. Take scoop of your bowel-cleansing formula in a tall glass of water.

**6:30 AM**
**EXERCISE**     Start with 5 minutes of rebounding, and work up to 15-20 minutes over time, or do exercise of your choice up to 30 minutes.

**7 AM**
**BREAKFAST**     (Drink a glass of water before eating): Take digestive enzymes and essential oil capsules with your meal.

**10 AM**     Take a scoop of your colon-cleansing formula in a glass of water, if needed.

**NOON**
**LUNCH**     (Drink a glass of water before eating): Take digestive enzymes and essential oil capsules with your meal.

**3 PM**     Take a scoop of your colon-cleansing formula in a glass of water, if needed.

**5 PM**     Optional short rebounding session (5-10 minutes) OR colon hydrotherapy session OR sauna or soak.

**7 PM**
**SUPPER**     (Drink a glass of water before eating): Take digestive enzymes and essential oil capsules with your meal.

**8:30 PM**     Optional time for soak, if desired.

**BEDTIME**     Take probiotic if not taken earlier in the day or if an extra dose is needed. If you missed a dose of your bowel-cleansing formula during the day, you may take it at this time.

**NOTE**     If you are not employed during the day, you may wish to do any of these therapies mid-morning instead of in a late afternoon time slot. The rebounding would ideally be done daily; the frequency of colonics will be based on the advice of your colon therapist; soaks or saunas may be done two to three times per week or as often as your healthcare professional recommends, working within the limits of your time constraints and financial considerations.

# NOTES
## on your cleansing experience

_____

_____

_____

_____

_____

_____

_____

_____

_____

_____

_____

_____

_____

_____

_____

_____

_____

_____

# Whole Body BASIC Cleanse

Once your colon is unclogged and working properly, you should be ready to tackle the herbal cleansing and detoxification of the whole body. Your ideal basic herbal cleansing program would consist of whole herbs. Such a product, formulated for people who have never cleansed before or who have not cleansed in a few years, would be a blend of safe, gentle and effective herbs that support all seven channels of elimination and provide gentle bowel stimulation. Such an herbal product will prepare your body for more advanced cleanses. It would be formulated in such a way as to alleviate the "cleansing reaction" symptoms that first-time cleansers may experience while cleansing, and would be comprised mostly of organic herbs.

Such a cleanse would come in two parts, one part to be taken in the morning and the second part in the evening. The morning formula would ideally consist of specific herbs to gently mobilize toxins stored in cells and tissues. The evening formula would contain basic herbs and a special blend of aromatic and stimulant herbs to assist in proper digestion. Such a formula promotes the safe elimination of these toxins from the body.

This basic cleanse (Part 1 plus Part II) would be a short one, approximately two weeks. Two Part I capsules would be taken in the morning before breakfast, then two Part II capsules in the evening before supper or at bedtime. Both would best be taken with eight ounces of water.

To integrate the Whole Body Basic Cleanse into your day, along with other supportive supplements and cleansing therapies, you will want to make yourself a cleansing schedule, as was suggested with the Focused Colon Cleanse. Your cleansing schedule for the basic cleanse described above will actually be very similar to the remaining cleanses described in this chapter. Most are two-part formulas, where two Part I capsules are taken in the morning and two Part II capsules are taken in the evening. Once again, a sample cleansing schedule is given, along with emphasis on the fact that this is only a suggested schedule. Please feel free to alter it to meet your personal schedule and needs.

This schedule incorporates other nutritional supplements that will enhance the cleansing process: **H**igh Fiber, Essential **O**ils, **P**robiotics and **E**nzymes (the **H.O.P.E.** formula).

## RECOMMENDED Whole Body BASIC Cleanse Part I Herbs

- Artichoke
- Blessed Thistle
- Burdock Root
- Dandelion
- Echinacea
- Fenugreek
- Garlic
- Green Tea
- Hawthorne Berry
- Horsetail
- Kelp
- Milk Thistle
- Mullein
- Nettle
- Oatstraw
- Oregano
- Parsley
- Red Clover
- Turmeric
- Wormwood
- Yarrow
- Yellow Dock

## RECOMMENDED Whole Body BASIC Cleanse Part II Herbs

- Buckthorn
- Flaxseed
- Rhubarb
- Marshmallow
- Slippery Elm
- Triphala

# SAMPLE
## Cleansing Schedule
(sample only, details may vary, according to your needs and schedule)

**6 AM** — Wake up. Take probiotic with a tall glass of water. Take Part I of Whole Body Basic Cleanse formula (2 capsules).

**6:30 AM EXERCISE** — Start with 5 minutes of rebounding, and work up to 15 to 20 minutes over time, or do exercise of your choice up to 30 minutes.

**7 AM BREAKFAST** — (Drink a glass of water before eating): Take digestive enzymes and essential oil capsules with your meal.

**10 AM** — Take 1-2 scoops of flax fiber (on an empty stomach) with a glass of water.

**NOON LUNCH** — (Drink a glass of water before eating); Take digestive enzymes and essential oil capsules with your meal.

**3 PM** — Take 1-2 scoops of flax fiber (on an empty stomach) with a glass of water.

**5 PM** — Take Part II of your Whole Body Basic Cleanse formula (2 capsules) with a glass of water.

**5:30 PM** — Optional short rebounding session (5-10 minutes) OR colon hydrotherapy session OR sauna or soak.

**7 PM SUPPER** — (Drink a glass of water before eating); Take digestive enzymes and essential oil capsules with your meal.

**8:30 PM** — Optional time for soak, if desired.

**BEDTIME** — Take fiber or probiotic if not taken during earlier in the day or if an extra dose is needed.

**NOTE** — If you are not employed during the day, you may wish to do any of these therapies mid-morning instead of in a late afternoon time slot. The rebounding would ideally be done daily; the frequency of colonics will be based on the advice of your colon therapist; soaks or saunas may be done two to three times per week or as often as your healthcare professional recommends, working within the limits of your time constraints and financial considerations.

# NOTES
## on your cleansing experience

_____

_____

_____

_____

_____

_____

_____

_____

_____

_____

_____

_____

_____

_____

_____

_____

_____

# Whole Body ADVANCED Cleanse

Your ideal advanced cleanse would be a blend of 22 herbs and minerals formulated for deep whole body cleansing. It would work more deeply than the Whole Body Basic Cleanse, pulling out wastes and toxins that are deeply imbedded in cells and tissues. In addition to cleansing the seven channels of elimination, the advanced cleanse would also provide them with nourishment and support, using powerful 4:1 and 5:1 herbal extracts (4 or 5 parts herb to one part liquid, such as alcohol/water). This cleanse would be longer than the Whole Body Basic Cleanse; it would be a 30-day, two-part program.

Part I of the advanced formula would be comprised of specially selected herbs that target each elimination organ of the body to mobilize wastes, moving them from tissues and organs into the lymphatic system and bloodstream. Once the toxins are in the blood and lymph, they are eliminated primarily through the kidneys (in urine) and the liver (in bile).

The herbs in Part I of the advanced formula function to:

• Mobilize wastes and toxins stored in tissues
• Stimulate bile flow in the liver for toxin excretion
• Protect the cells of the liver from the effects of chemical toxins
• Cleanse the urinary tract
• Stimulate lymphatic flow
• Boost immune function
• Decrease respiratory mucus
• Benefit skin conditions
• Purify the blood

Part II, of the advanced formula would ideally contain magnesium hydroxide. Magnesium draws fluids from the bowel wall into the lumen (open space in the colon). It therefore has laxative properties.

The herbs contained in the Part II function to:

• Tone and strengthen the bowel
• Soothe bowel irritation
• Lubricate the bowel
• Decrease bowel mucus
• Stimulate bowel movements for elimination of liver, digestive and bowel toxins

It would be best to take two Part I capsules of this advanced formula with 8 oz. of water every morning upon rising and two Part II capsules every evening (an hour before dinner or at bedtime) with 8 oz. of water for 30 days. This protocol may be followed several times per year for optimal results. Depending upon your state of health, you may experience a range of results while taking this advanced formula, from weight loss and increased bowel movements to cold and flu-like symptoms. If such cleansing symptoms occur, temporarily reduce dose to one capsule of Parts I and II per day for a few days, and then resume full dosage in a few days.

The sample cleansing schedule incorporates the above cleanse. This schedule incorporates other nutritional supplements that will enhance the cleansing process: **H**igh Fiber, Essential **O**ils, **P**robiotics and **E**nzymes (the **H.O.P.E.** formula).

## RECOMMENDED Whole Body ADVANCED Cleanse Part I Herbs

• Artichoke
• Ashwaganda
• Beet
• Burdock Root
• Bupleurum
• Celandine
• Chlorella
• Corn Silk
• Dandelion
• Hawthorne Berry
• Larch
• Mullein
• Milk Thistle
• Red Clover
• Turmeric

## RECOMMENDED Whole Body ADVANCED Cleanse Part II Herbs

• Magnesium Hydroxide
• Cape Aloe
• Rhubarb
• Slippery Elm
• Marshmallow
• Fennel
• Ginger
• Triphala

# SAMPLE
## Cleansing Schedule
(sample only, details may vary, according to your needs and schedule)

**6 AM** — Wake up. Take probiotic with a tall glass of water. Take Part I of your Whole Body Advanced Cleanse (2 capsules).

**6:30 AM EXERCISE** — Start with 5 minutes of rebounding, and work up to 15-20 minutes over time, or do exercise of your choice up to 30 minutes.

**7 AM BREAKFAST** — (Drink a glass of water before eating): Take digestive enzymes and essential oil capsules with your meal.

**10 AM** — Take 1-2 scoops of flax fiber (on an empty stomach) with a glass of water.

**NOON LUNCH** — (Drink a glass of water before eating): Take digestive enzymes and essential oil capsules with your meal.

**3 PM** — Take 1-2 scoops of flax fiber (on an empty stomach) with a glass of water.

**5 PM** — Take Part II of your Whole Body Advanced Cleanse (2 capsules) with a glass of water.

**5:30 PM** — Optional short rebounding session (5-10 minutes) OR colon hydrotherapy session OR sauna or soak.

**7 PM SUPPER** — (Drink a glass of water before eating): Take digestive enzymes and essential oil capsules with your meal.

**8:30 PM** — Optional time for soak, if desired.

**BEDTIME** — Take fiber or probiotic if not taken earlier in the day or if an extra dose is needed.

**NOTE** — If you are not employed during the day, you may wish to do any of these therapies mid-morning instead of in a late afternoon time slot. The rebounding would ideally be done daily; the frequency of colonics will be based on the advice of your colon therapist; soaks or saunas may be done two to three times per week or as often as your healthcare professional recommends, working within the limits of your time constraints and financial considerations.

# NOTES
## on your cleansing experience

_____

_____

_____

_____

_____

_____

_____

_____

_____

_____

_____

_____

_____

_____

_____

_____

_____

_____

_____

_____

_____

# Whole Body MAINTENANCE Cleanse

We're exposed to toxins everyday, but aren't always ingesting the nutrients necessary to break them down and eliminate them. An effective maintenance formula would be designed to fill this nutritional gap. It would provide important nutrients and antioxidants (in vegetable, rather than animal-based, capsules) that support normal detoxification mechanisms and protect the body from the health-damaging effects of chemicals and biological toxins. Such a maintenance formula may be considered the multi-vitamin of cleansing. Though powerful, it is gentle enough to be taken every day to insure the health of the body.

Your ideal maintenance formula would be made with organic whole herbs (not high-potency extracts) and a wide range of nutraceuticals (compounds isolated from food that are used for their health benefits) to support daily detoxification and optimize daily health. It also would contain the same blend of nine herbs and cellulase (to maximize absorption of whole herbs) found in your Whole Body Basic Cleanse. The recommended herbs in such a maintenance formula have general benefits and support normal physiological activities, rather than initiating a profound cleansing response.

Like your basic and advanced cleanses, your maintenance cleanse would ideally contain herbs that support all seven channels of elimination.

The herbs and nutraceuticals in the maintenance formula would ideally:

• Provide antioxidant protection
• Protect the liver from toxins
• Inhibit re-absorption of toxins in bile
• Support liver detoxification
• Boost immune function
• Strengthen blood vessels

Take two capsules of the Whole Body Maintenance Cleanse herbal formula in the morning upon rising and two capsules one hour before supper or at bedtime. Be sure and drink 8 oz. of water with the capsules.

As with the other cleanses, you may wish to write out a cleansing schedule that meets your needs. This schedule incorporates other nutritional supplements that will enhance the cleansing process: **H**igh Fiber, Essential **O**ils, **P**robiotics and **E**nzymes (the **H.O.P.E.** formula).

## RECOMMENDED MAINTENANCE Cleanse Herbs & Nutraceuticals

### HERBS

• Artichoke
• Dandelion
• Fenugreek
• Garlic
• Green Tea
• Marshmallow
• Milk Thistle
• Mullein
• Nettle

• Oatstraw
• Oregano
• Parsley
• Red Clover
• Slippery Elm
• Spirulina
• Triphala
• Tumeric

### NUTRACEUTICALS

• Alpha Lipoic Acid
• Coenzyme Q-10
• Gamma Oryzanol
• L-Glutamine
• L-Glutathione
• Lutein

• Lycopene
• MSM
• N-Acetyl-Cysteine
• Resveratrol
• Quercetin
• Zeaxanthin

# SAMPLE
## Cleansing Schedule
(sample only, details may vary, according to your needs and schedule)

| | |
|---|---|
| **6 AM** | Wake up. Take probiotic with a tall glass of water. Take 2 capsules of your Whole Body Maintenance Cleanse herbal formula. |
| **6:30 AM**<br>**EXERCISE** | Start with 5 minutes of rebounding, and work up to 15-20 minutes over time, or do exercise of your choice up to 30 minutes. |
| **7 AM**<br>**BREAKFAST** | (Drink a glass of water before eating): Take digestive enzymes and essential oil capsules with your meal. |
| **10 AM** | Take 1-2 scoops of flax fiber (on an empty stomach) with a glass of water. |
| **NOON**<br>**LUNCH** | (Drink a glass of water before eating): Take digestive enzymes and essential oil capsules with your meal. |
| **3 PM** | Take 1-2 scoops of flax fiber (on an empty stomach) with a glass of water. |
| **5 PM** | Take 2 capsules of your Whole Body Maintenance Cleanse herbal formula with a glass of water. |
| **5:30 PM** | Optional short rebounding session (5-10 minutes) OR colon hydrotherapy session OR sauna or soak. |
| **7 PM**<br>**SUPPER** | (Drink a glass of water before eating): Take digestive enzymes and essential oil capsules with your meal. |
| **8:30 PM** | Optional time for soak, if desired. |
| **BEDTIME** | Take fiber or probiotic if not taken during earlier in the day or if an extra dose is needed. |
| **NOTE** | If you are not employed during the day, you may wish to do any of these therapies mid-morning instead of in a late afternoon time slot. The rebounding would ideally be done daily; the frequency of colonics will be based on the advice of your colon therapist; soaks or saunas may be done two to three times per week or as often as your healthcare professional recommends, working within the limits of your time constraints and financial considerations. |

# NOTES
## on your cleansing experience

# Focused LIVER Cleanse

We have already noted in Chapter 4, Channels of Elimination, that the body's major detoxification organ, the liver, employs a two-part detoxification system that is dependent upon specific nutrients. When these nutrients are lacking or are in short supply and toxic exposure is high, toxins overwhelm the body, and the stage is set for illness to develop. For many people, liver damage from alcohol, prescription or recreational drugs, hepatitis and repeated or acute toxic exposures, has created a need for extra liver support. Those with liver issues can benefit greatly from use of an herbal liver-cleansing product. Ideally, such a product would contain a blend of specific herbs, antioxidants and nutraceuticals known to support, protect, stimulate and detoxify the liver. Such a product may be taken by anyone who simply wants to maximize liver support. It may be taken on an ongoing basis, along with other herbal cleanses to maximize liver function.

The ideal herbal liver-cleansing product would supply many of the necessary nutrients for Phase 1 and Phase 2 liver detoxification pathways, and contain nutraceuticals that:

• Provide the necessary nutrients for both phases of liver detoxification
• Protect the liver from chemical toxins
• Provide antioxidants
• Stimulate bile production
• Provide important liver antioxidants and their precursors

The recommended herbs in this ideal liver-cleansing product would:

• Stimulate bile flow to enhance elimination of toxins
• Cleanse the kidneys for safe toxin elimination
• Support the liver in dealing with chemical toxins
• Scavenge free radicals

Two Part I capsules of the recommended liver-cleansing formula would be taken in the morning with water before breakfast. It would contain nutraceuticals, herbs and antioxidants vital to support Phase 1 and Phase 2 detoxification.

Part II of your herbal liver-cleansing formula would ideally contain important Indian herbs long used in Ayurvedic medicine. These herbs have liver-protecting and detoxification properties that have been documented in scientific studies. Two Part II capsules would be taken at night with water before bed.

Provided once again is a sample cleansing schedule which incorporates other nutritional supplements that will enhance the cleansing process: **H**igh Fiber, Essential **O**ils, **P**robiotics and **E**nzymes (the **H.O.P.E.** formula).

## RECOMMENDED LIVER Cleansing Formula Part I Herbs

• Alpha Lipoic Acid
• Artichoke
• Dandelion
• Green Tea
• L-Methionine
• L-Taurine
• Milk Thistle
• N-Acetyl-Cysteine
• Phosphatidyl-choline
• Selenuim
• Turmeric

## RECOMMENDED LIVER Cleansing Formula Part II Herbs

• Andrographis paniculata
• Belleric myrobalan
• Boerhavia diffusa
• Eclipta alba
• Picrorhiza kurroa
• Tinospora cordifolia

# SAMPLE
## Cleansing Schedule
(sample only, details may vary, according to your needs and schedule)

**6 AM**    Wake up. Take probiotic with a tall glass of water. Take Part I of your Focused Liver Cleanse (2 capsules).

**6:30 AM EXERCISE**    Start with 5 minutes of rebounding, and work up to 15-20 minutes over time, or do exercise of your choice up to 30 minutes.

**7 AM BREAKFAST**    (Drink a glass of water before eating): Take digestive enzymes and essential oil capsules with your meal.

**10 AM**    Take 1-2 scoops of flax fiber (on an empty stomach) with a glass of water.

**NOON LUNCH**    (Drink a glass of water before eating): Take digestive enzymes and essential oil capsules with your meal.

**3 PM**    Take 1-2 scoops of flax fiber (on an empty stomach) with a glass of water.

**5 PM**    Take Part II of your Focused Liver Cleanse (2 capsules) with a glass of water.

**5:30 PM**    Optional short rebounding session (5-10 minutes) OR colon hydrotherapy session OR sauna or soak.

**7 PM SUPPER**    (Drink a glass of water before eating); Take digestive enzymes and essential oil capsules with your meal.

**8:30 PM**    Optional time for soak, if desired.

**BEDTIME**    Take fiber or probiotic if not taken during earlier in the day or if an extra dose is needed.

**NOTE**    If you are not employed during the day, you may wish to do any of these therapies mid-morning instead of in a late afternoon time slot. The rebounding would ideally be done daily; the frequency of colonics will be based on the advice of your colon therapist; soaks or saunas may be done two to three times per week as often as your healthcare professional recommends, working within the limits of your time constraints and financial considerations.

# NOTES
## on your cleansing experience

_____
_____
_____
_____
_____
_____
_____
_____
_____
_____
_____
_____
_____
_____
_____
_____

## Focused HEAVY METAL Cleanse

Anyone living in the 21st century has significant heavy metal exposure from sources outlined in Chapter 1. Heavy metals are among the most damaging pollutants affecting us today, and they are also some of the most difficult toxins to eliminate from the body. Progressive medical doctors have long used a process known as *chelation* to coax heavy metals out of the body. Chelation involves the introduction into the bloodstream of a substance that attracts the metals. Metals attach to this "chelating agent." Some nutrients serve as effective chelating agents when taken orally.

An increase of heavy metals in the body will displace needed nutritive minerals, possibly leading to deficiencies. It is therefore necessary to include key nutritive minerals when undergoing a Focused Heavy Metal Cleanse. The ideal heavy metal cleansing product would be a two-part formula containing key nutrients to restore normal metabolic processes that have been disturbed by heavy metal toxicity and important botanicals and nutrients that bind and help excrete heavy metals from the body.

Two Part I capsules of the Focused Heavy Metal Cleanse herbal formula would be taken in the morning with breakfast, with water. This would ideally supply balanced amounts of key minerals, replacing those minerals that might become displaced or imbalanced from heavy metal toxicity and through the chelation process itself. Two Part II capsules of the Focused Heavy Metal Cleanse would be taken in the evening before dinner or at bedtime, with water. Ideally, this would contain the ingredients to bind and excrete heavy metals from the body.

A heavy metal cleansing product such as that described above would support the elimination of heavy metals without losing vital nutrients in the process. It would ideally be delivered in vegetable capsules and contain no binders or fillers.

The cleansing schedule on the opposite page, is a sample that incorporates the Focused Heavy Metal Cleanse with other elements of your detoxification program: **H**igh Fiber, Essential **O**ils, **P**robiotics and **E**nzymes (the **H.O.P.E.** formula).

### RECOMMENDED HEAVY METAL Cleansing Formula Part I Herbs

- Biotin
- Boron
- Calcium
- Chromium
- Copper
- Folic Acid
- Manganese
- Magnesium
- Molybdenum
- Selenium
- Vanadium
- Vitamin C
- Vitamin B-1
- Vitamin B-2
- Vitamin B-3
- Vitamin B-6
- Vitamin B-5
- Vitamin B-12
- Zinc

### RECOMMENDED HEAVY METAL Cleansing Formula Part II Herbs

- Alpha Lipoic Acid
- Bladderwrack
- Chlorella
- Cilantro
- Garlic
- Kelp
- L-Leucine
- N-Acetyl-Cysteine
- Sodium Alginate
- Spirulina

# SAMPLE
## Cleansing Schedule
(sample only, details may vary, according to your needs and schedule)

| | |
|---|---|
| **6 AM** | Wake up. Take probiotic with a tall glass of water. |
| **6:30 AM EXERCISE** | Start with 5 minutes of rebounding, and work up to 15-20 minutes over time, or do exercise of your choice up to 30 minutes. |
| **7 AM BREAKFAST** | (Drink a glass of water before eating): Take digestive enzymes and essential oil capsules with your meal. |
| | Take two Part I capsules of your Focused Heavy Metal Cleanse WITH breakfast. |
| **10 AM** | Take 1-2 scoops of flax fiber (on an empty stomach) with a glass of water. |
| **NOON LUNCH** | (Drink a glass of water before eating): Take digestive enzymes and essential oil capsules with your meal. |
| **3 PM** | Take 1-2 scoops of flax fiber (on an empty stomach) with a glass of water. |
| **5 PM** | Take two Part II capsules of your Focused Heavy Metal Cleanse with a glass of water. |
| **5:30 PM** | Optional short rebounding session (5-10 minutes) OR colon hydrotherapy session OR sauna or soak. |
| **7 PM SUPPER** | (Drink a glass of water before eating): Take digestive enzymes and essential oil capsules with your meal. |
| **8:30 PM** | Optional time for soak, if desired. |
| **BEDTIME** | Take fiber or probiotic if not taken during earlier in the day or if an extra dose is needed. |

**NOTE** If you are not employed during the day, you may wish to do any of these therapies mid-morning instead of in a late afternoon time slot. The rebounding would ideally be done daily; the frequency of colonics will be based on the advice of your colon therapist; soaks or saunas may be done two to three times per week or as often as your healthcare professional recommends, working within the limits of your time constraints and financial considerations.

# NOTES
## on your cleansing experience

_____

_____

_____

_____

_____

_____

_____

_____

_____

_____

_____

_____

_____

_____

_____

_____

_____

_____

# The Steps to Internal Health

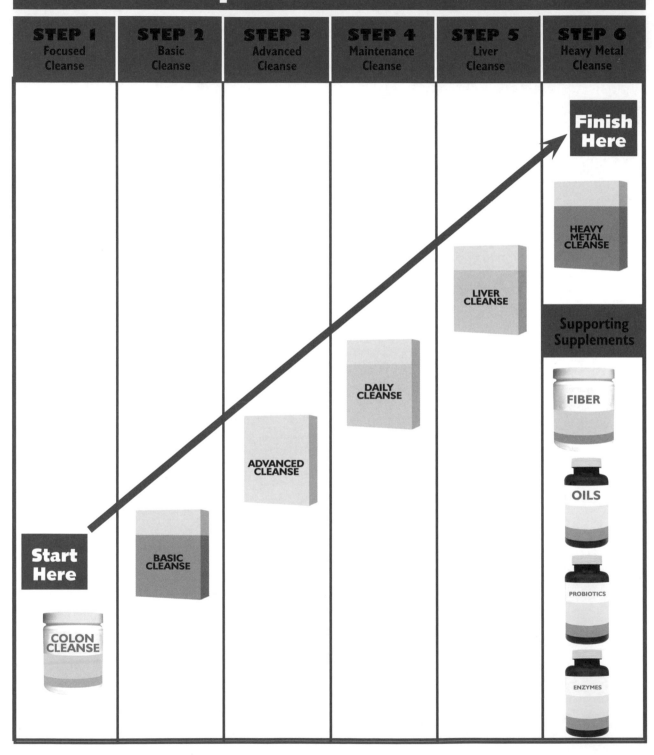

| STEP 1 Focused Cleanse | STEP 2 Basic Cleanse | STEP 3 Advanced Cleanse | STEP 4 Maintenance Cleanse | STEP 5 Liver Cleanse | STEP 6 Heavy Metal Cleanse |
|---|---|---|---|---|---|

Finish Here

HEAVY METAL CLEANSE

LIVER CLEANSE

DAILY CLEANSE

ADVANCED CLEANSE

Supporting Supplements

FIBER

OILS

PROBIOTICS

Start Here

BASIC CLEANSE

ENZYMES

COLON CLEANSE

# Oil and Fiber Too!

In addition to the dietary and lifestyle changes and herbal/nutraceutical cleanses outlined here, it is also highly recommended that extra fiber and essential fatty acids be consumed during any cleanse to support the detoxification process.

Look for a source of omega-3, -6 and -9 essential fatty acids from flax, fish and borage oils, ideally one that also contains lipase, the enzyme needed to break down those oils. The added lipase will also help keep the taste of the fish oil from repeating. The oils in such a product help lubricate the intestines to ensure smooth and gentle elimination. These oils not only provide the colon with the lubrication it needs to eliminate waste two to three times per day, but they also give the body the essential fatty acids vital to many cellular functions, and hence good health. Such an oil product should be taken with all cleansing and maintenance formulas. It will be especially helpful to those with dry skin and/or skin conditions, digestive distress, menstrual and pre-menstrual disturbances, and conditions of the joints and tendons.

A flax fiber supplement is an important addition to any cleansing program. Fiber has been shown to aid elimination through the bowel and absorb toxins in the intestine, preventing their re-absorption. Look for a flax fiber product that not only binds toxic material and escorts it from the body, but also contains natural ingredients like probiotics and L-glutamine to support the health of the digestive system, and herbs like slippery elm, marshmallow and triphala to soothe and lubricate the bowel.

Another kind of fiber would contain organic flax, acacia and oat bran fibers. This would be an organic triple fiber blend which would also aid elimination and absorb toxins in the intestine.

## RECOMMENDED READING

*Beyond Amalgam: The Hidden Health Hazard Posed by Jawbone Cavitations* by Suzin Stockton, Power of One Publishing, 2000.

*Detoxify or Die* by Sherry A. Rogers, MD, Sand Key Company, Inc., 2002.

*Excitotoxins: The Taste that Kills* by Russell L. Blaylock, Health Press, 1997.

*Home Safe Home* by Debra Lynn Dadd, Tarcher/Penguin, 2005.

*Mold Warriors* by Ritchie C. Shoemaker, MD, Gateway Press, Inc., 2005.

*Our Toxic World: A Wake Up Call* by Doris J. Rapp, MD, Environmental Medical Research Foundation, 2003.

*Surviving the Toxic Crisis* by Dr. William R. Kellas and Dr. Andrea Sharon Dworkin, Professional Preference, 1996.

*Sweet Poison: How the World's Most Popular Artificial Sweetener is Killing Us — My Story* by Janet Starr Hull, New Horizon Press, 2001.

*The Crazy Makers: How the Food Industry is Destroying Our Brains and Harming Our Children* by Carol Simontacchi, Jeremy P. Tarcher, 2001.

*The Fluoride Deception* by Christopher Bryson, Seven Stories Press, 2004.

*The Mold Survival Guide for Your Home and For Your Health* by Jeffrey C. May and Connie L. May, Johns Hopkins University Press, 2004.

*The Paleo Diet* by Loren Cordain, Ph.D., John Wiley and Sons, Inc., 2002.

*Tooth Truth* by Frank Jerome, New Century Press, 2000.

# Essential Cleansing
## for Perfect Health

# APPENDIX

# Endnotes

## INTRODUCTION

1   http://dictionary.cambridge.org/define.asp?key=toxic*1+0&dict=A

2   Ibid.

3   http://dictionary.cambridge.org/define.asp?key=poison*1+0&dict=A

4   Stedman's Concise Medical Dictionary, 4th Edition, Lippincott Williams & Wilkins, 2001, p. 999.

5   William Randall Kellas, Ph.D. and Andrea Sharon Dworkin, N.D., Surviving the Toxic Crisis, Professional Preference, 1996, p. 1.

## CHAPTER 1

1   T. Woodruff, J. Grillo, K. Schoendorf, "The Relationship Between Selected Causes of Post-neonatal Infant Mortality and Particulate Air Pollution in the United States," Environmental Health Perspective, June 1997, 105(6).

2   Dr. James H. Martin, Health Alert (e-bulletin), April 26, 2004 (information taken, in part, from Carol Simontachhihi's book, The Crazy Makers: How the Food Industry is Destroying Our Brains and Harming Our Children).

3   Ibid.

4   Paula DiPerna, Environmental Hazards to Children Public Affairs Pamphlet, 1981

5   http://www.nci.nih.gov/newscenter/benchmarks-vol4-issue3/page1 (Nancy Nelson, "The Majority of Cancers are Linked to the Environment," June 17, 2004.)

6   Sherry A. Rogers, MD, Detoxify or Die, Sand Key Company, Inc., 2002, p. 30.

7   Ibid.

8   http://www.ewg.org/reports/bodyburden/findings.php

9   Neurotoxicology, 2002 Sep; 23(3): 329-39 (as cited in Power Point by Alex Vasquez, DC, ND for the Institute for Functional Medicine, 2004)

10  Doris J. Rapp, MD, Our Toxic World: A Wake Up Call, Environmental Medical Research Foundation, 2003, back cover.

11  http://www.idph.state.il.us/envhealth/factsheets/polychlorinatedbiphenyls.htm

12  http://www.ecy.wa.gov/programs/hwtr/demodebris/pages2/pcbsummary.html

13  Dr. James H. Martin, Health Alert, November 9, 2004 (reported source: Frederick Vom Saal, an endocrinologist at the University of Missouri at Colombia)

14  Rapp, Op. Cit.

15  Dr. James H. Martin, Health Alert, September 17, 2004 (reported source: Andy Coghlan, NewScientist.com, 9-8-04)

16  Rapp, Op. Cit.

17  Dr. James H. Martin, Health Alert, November 29, 2004 (reported source: Dr. Martin's How Toxic Are You? Workshop)

18  The Globe and Mail, Friday, May 21, 2004, p. A17 (as cited in Power Point by Alex Vasquez, DC, ND for the Institute for Functional Medicine, 2004)

19  http://www.panna.org/campaigns/docsrespass/chemicalTrespass2004.dv.html (as cited in Power Point by Alex Vasquez, DC, ND for the Institute for Functional Medicine, 2004)

20  Dr. James H. Martin, Health Alert, April 26, 2004, Op. Cit.

21  Ibid.

22  Exp Neurol. 1998 Apr; 150(2): 339-42 (as cited in Power Point by Alex Vasquez, DC, ND for the Institute for Functional Medicine, 2004)

23  J Clin Endocrinol Metab. 2004 Sep; 89(9): 4665-72 (as cited in Power Point by Alex Vasquez, DC, ND for the Institute for Functional Medicine, 2004)

24  Environ Health Perspect. 2002 Sep; 110(9): 853-8 (as cited in Power Point by Alex Vasquez, DC, ND for the Institute for Functional Medicine, 2004)

25  Power Point presentation by Alex Vasquez, DC, ND for the Institute for Functional Medicine, 2004

26  Rapp, Op. Cit., p. 4.

27  William Randall Kellas, PhD and Andrea Sharon Dworkin, ND, Surviving the Toxic Crisis, Professional Preference, 1996, p. 176-177.

28  Michael Murray, ND and Joseph Pizzorno, ND, Encyclopedia of Natural Medicine, Revised 2nd Edition, Prima Health, 1998, p. 105.

29  ACCM Health Sense (Newsletter), Vol. X, Issue 8, August 2004.

30  Dr. James H. Martin, Health Alert, November 29, 2004 (reported source: Dr. Martin's How Toxic Are You? Workshop)

31  Doris J. Rapp, MD, Our Toxic World: A Wake Up Call, p. 237-238

32  Suzin Stockton, The Terrain is Everything, Power of One Publishing, 2000, p. 50.

33  www.indoorpollution.com

34  Ibid.

35  Stockton, op. cit., p. 128.

36  Ibid, p. 129.

37  Ibid., p. 128.

38  http://www.askoxford.com/concise_oed/outgas?view=uk

39  Drs. William R. Kellas and Andrea Sharon Dworkin, Surviving the Toxic Crisis, p74 (quoted from Chemical Exposures:Low Levels: High Stakes)

40  Kellas and Dworkin, Op. cit., p. 75.

41  Ibid.

42  Ibid, p. 74 (quoted from Neurotoxins: At Home and the Workplace, Report by the Committee on Science and Technology, U.S. House of Representatives, Sept. 16, 1986, Report 99-827)

43  Barry Groves, Fluoride: Drinking Ourselves to Death, Newleaf, 2001, p.

1.  (quoted from Clinical Toxicology of Commercial Products, 5th Edition, 1984.)

44  www.mercola.com/fcfi/pf/2004/dec/25/washing_hair.htm

45  Ibid.

46  http://www.epa.gov/iaq/voc.html

47  http://www.epa.gov/iaq/formalde.html

48  Stockton, Op. Cit., p. 136.

49  Ibid, p. 135.

50  Ibid.

51  Jeffrey C. May and Connie L. May, The Mold Survival Guide for Your Home and for Your Health, The Johns Hopkins University Press, 2004, p. 4.

52  Ibid, p. 50.

53  http://www.mercola.com/fcgi/pf/2005/feb/19/common_toxins.htm

54  http://www.indoorpollution.com/mold_health_problem.htm

55  http://greatdayamerica.com/health/preventative/innowave6.shtml

56  Stockton, Op. Cit., p. 184-185.

57  Brenda Watson, Renew Your Life, Renew Life Press and Information Services, 2002, p. 34.

58  Stockton, Op. Cit., p. 185.

59  http://4optimallife.com/Dangers-Of-Chlorine-To-Your-Health.html  (quoted from Dr Z Rona MD MSc)

60  http://www.newmediaexplorer.org/sepp/Death%20by%20Medicine%20Nov%2027.doc

61  Ibid.

62  Melissa Palmer, MD, Hepatitis Liver Disease: What You Need to Know, Avery Publishing Group, 2000, p. 377.

63  www.healthcarealternatives.net (article: Jawbone Cavitations: Infarction, Infection & Systemic Disease by Suzin Stockton MA – 2002)

## CHAPTER 2

1  Brenda Watson, Renew Your Life, Renew Life Press and Information Services, 2002, p. 18.

2  Ibid, p. 21.

3  http://healthyfutures.net/PatScardina/products/catalog/probiotics-info.php

## CHAPTER 3

1  http://www.liverdoctor.com/03_detoxpathways.asp

2  Ibid.

3  Jack Tips, PhD, Your Liver … Your Lifeline, Apple-A-Day-Press, 1993, p. 25.

4  www.liverdoctor.com/Section2/08_symptoms.asp

5  Op.Cit., Tips, p.76-84.

6  Matthias Rath, MD, Why Animals Don't Get Heart Attacks…But People Do, Dr. Rath Health Foundation, 2003, p.57.

7  Ibid, p. 80.

8  www.chiroweb.com/archives/14/10/03.html

9  Ibid.

## CHAPTER 5

1  http://www.infoholix.net/category.php?mId=58

2  Phyllis A. Balch, CNC and James F. Balch, MD,

Prescription for Nutritional Healing, Third Edition, Avery, 2000, p. 708.

3   Jacqueline Krohn, MD, and Frances Taylor, MA, Natural Detoxification: A Practical Encyclopedia, Hartly and Marks Publishers, 2000, p. 407.

4   Bettman, Otto L., Ph.D., A Pictorial History of Medicine, Charles C. Thomas, Publisher, 1956, page. 3.

5   www.optimalhealthnetwork.com/tek9. asp?pg=Weight

6   Hal Huggins, DDS, Detoxification, Peak Energy Performance, p. 19.

7   Sherry A. Rogers, MD, Detoxify or Die, Sand Key Company, Inc., 2002, p. 194.

8   Cheryl Townsley, Cleansing Made Simple, LRH Publishing, 1997, p. 47-48.

9   Ibid, p. 23.

10   Dr. William R. Kellas and Dr. Andrea Sharon Dworkin, Thriving in a Toxic World, Professional Preference, 1996, p. 372-373.

11   Ibid. p. 373-374.

## CHAPTER 6

1   Stedman's Concise Medical Dictionary for the Health Professions, 4th Edition, Lippincott Williams and Wilkins, 2001, p.113.

# Ingredient Reference

## HERBS

**Acacia Gum** – Acacia comes from the gum of the acacia tree. As well as its properties as a fiber supplement, it is also a 'prebiotic', which means that it increases good gut flora (the friendly bacteria in the gut). It slows down colonic fermentation, which decreases gas and bloating. Acacia gum is also considered a demulcent, which soothes irritated or inflamed mucous tissue.

**Andrographis paniculata** — Used traditionally in dyspepsia, dysentery, liver disease, intestinal parasites, hemorrhoids, fever, upper respiratory tract infection, cough, bronchitis, pruritus (severe itching), inflammatory skin conditions, leprosy, intense thirst, burning sensations, wounds, ulcers and acute and chronic malaria.

**Artichoke Leaf** — Stimulates bile flow, protects liver against toxic damage, helps lower high cholesterol; used traditionally in dyspepsia (indigestion), liver/gallbladder problems and dyslipidemia (lipoprotein metabolism disorder).

**Ashwaganda Root** — Used traditionally for weakness and fatigue, lung problems, joint pain, mental disorders, insomnia, infertility and cancer; helps regulate the adrenal glands.

**Beet Leaf** — Used traditionally for constipation and toxicity; helps reduce damaging fats from the liver.

**Belleric Myrobalan** — Used traditionally for nausea, diarrhea, hemorrhage, cough, asthma, fever, prolapsed organs, bladder stones, weakness, eye diseases.

**Black Pepper** — Stimulates secretion of saliva/gastric mucus.

**Bladderwrack** — A sea vegetable used traditionally for hypothyroidism, goiter, obesity, cystitis, heart disease, rheumatism, leucorrhea (vaginal discharge), lymphatic congestion and cancer. It is a chelating agent that provides immune support.

**Blessed Thistle** — Used traditionally for poor digestion, colic, diarrhea, the common cold, intermittent fever, dysmenorrhea (painful periods), and deficient lactation.

**Boerhavia diffusa** — Used traditionally for dyspepsia, gastritis, ulcers, constipation, intestinal parasites, jaundice, cirrhosis, bronchitis, asthma, cystitis, kidney diseases, muscle and joint pain, leucorrhea (vaginal discharge), dysmenorrhea (painful periods), heart disease, anemia, epilepsy and weakness.

**Buckthorn** — Traditionally used for indigestion, liver/gallbladder problems, constipation, hemorrhoids, joint pain and cancer.

**Bupleurum Root** — Used traditionally for dyspepsia, ulcers, liver/gallbladder problems, joint pain, irregular menstruation and cancer; has anti-viral properties.

**Burdock Root** — Used traditionally for skin diseases, liver/gallbladder problems, constipation, joint pain and dyslipidemia (lipoprotein metabolism disorder).

**Cape Aloe Gel/Latex** — This mild laxative is used traditionally for irritable bowel, ulcerations, constipation, intestinal parasites, wounds and burns.

**Cayenne** — Increases blood flow to the intestines; works as a catalyst, helping other ingredients get into the bloodstream faster.

**Celandine Leaf** — Used traditionally for liver/gallbladder pain, jaundice, hemorrhoids, skin diseases, migraines and fungal infections.

**Chlorella** — Used traditionally for cancer, immune deficiency, chronic infection, heavy metal toxicity, radiation poisoning, hepatitis and pancreatitis; a blood purifier.

**Cilantro** —Also known as Chinese parsley. It has been used traditionally for dyspepsia, heavy metal toxicity, skin diseases and burning sensations. Cilantro mobilizes metals to move them from the tissue.

**Cinnamon** — One of the oldest herbal medicines known. It has been used traditionally to treat all types of infections, sore throats, colds, coughs, indigestion, diarrhea, flatulence, arthritis, bad breath and menstrual cramps.

**Coriander** — Stimulates gastric juices, reduces spasms.

**Corn Silk** — Used traditionally for urinary tract irritation and cystitis; a diuretic to flush the kidneys.

**Cumin** — Relieves gas in the stomach and intestines; relieves diarrhea.

**Dandelion Leaf** — Traditionally used for edema (water retention), enuresis (bedwetting), incontinence, kidney stones, skin disease, liver/gallbladder problems, cardiac arrhythmia, potassium depletion and oral rehydration.

**Dandelion Root** — Traditionally used for skin diseases, liver/gallbladder problems, constipation and dysmenorrhea (painful periods); stimulates bile; a gentle laxative.

**Echinacea Root** — Traditionally used for acute fever, sinus congestion, lymphatic congestion, pharyngitis (inflammation of the throat or pharynx), bronchitis, infection, abdominal pain, skin disease, cancer, acute injuries, bites, stings and immunodeficiency.

**Eclipta alba** — Used traditionally for dyspepsia, hemorrhoids, hepatosplenomegaly (enlargement of spleen and liver), cholelithiasis (production of gallstones), jaundice, cirrhosis, bronchitis, asthma, skin diseases, ophthalmia (severe eye inflammation), premature graying, alopecia (falling hair), edema (water retention), anemia, mental disorders, menorrhagia (long, heavy periods), fatigue and insect and snake bites.

**Fennel Seed** — This is a carminative herb, which prevents griping, stimulates gastrointestinal motility and reduces bloating and gas.

**Fenugreek** — Used traditionally for poor digestion, constipation, ulcers, bowel inflammation, joint pain, skin diseases, weight loss, coughs, bronchitis, infertility and deficient lactation.

**Flax seed** — Traditionally used for constipation, dry skin, mucosal irritation, dyslipidemia (a disorder of lipoprotein metabolism, including lipoprotein overproduction or deficiency) and weight management.

**Garlic** — Used traditionally for colds and flu, coughs, bronchitis, pertussis (whooping cough), pneumonia, candidiasis, intestinal parasites, bacteria infections, hyperlipidemia, artherosclerosis, cancer, immune deficiency and weakness.

**Gentian** — Considered a bitter; stimulates digestive juices.

**Ginger Root** — Stimulates digestion, saliva, gastric juices and bile.

**Green Tea Extract** — a concentrated extract from unfermented tea (Camellia sinensis) leaves, a popular beverage in East Asia. Its regular consumption is associated with a decreased incidence of several different cancers. The extract is a potent source of polyphenols (antioxidant chemicals that give some plants their color and may protect against some common health problems and possibly certain effects of aging). These chemical compounds have been shown to inhibit tumor development and reduce free radical activity.

**Hawthorne Berry** — Used traditionally for heart disease, atherosclerosis, hypertension (high blood pressure) and chronic injuries.

**Horsetail** — Traditionally used for arthritis, musculoskeletal injury, hay fever, tuberculosis, bladder infection and irritation, incontinence, edema, renal calculi (kidney stones), menorrhagia (long, heavy periods) and intestinal hemorrhage.

**Kelp** — Used traditionally for hypothyroidism (underactive thyroid), goiter (enlarged thyroid), obesity, cystitis (inflammation of the urinary bladder), heart disease, rheumatism, leucorrhea (vaginal discharge), lymphatic congestion and cancer.

**Larch Gum** — Used traditionally for the common cold, constipation, liver disease, immune deficiency and cancer; cleans out the lymphatic system.

**Marshmallow** — Traditionally used for mucosal irritation and inflammation, wasting diseases, external wounds and immune dysfunction.

**Milk Thistle Seed** — Used traditionally for liver/gallbladder problems, liver damage and deficient lactation; strengthens the walls of liver cells, making them less susceptible to invasion by viruses.

**Mullein Leaf** — Used traditionally for the common cold, bronchitis, asthma, pleurisy and wounds; increases blood flow to lungs.

**Nettle Leaf** — Traditionally used for anemia, weakness, nutrient deficiency, skin disease, bronchitis, asthma, hay fever, arthritis, osteoporosis, sports injuries, menorrhagia (long, heavy periods), bladder irritability and kidney/bladder stones.

**Oat Fiber** — A soluble dietary fiber that is known for lowering the risk of heart disease by reducing blood cholesterol levels and for helping regulate blood sugar levels. One clinical study reported that beta-glucan (a sugar-molecule string) from oat fiber promoted healthy bile acid secretion, which can help combat constipation and remove toxins from the body. It has also been found that "Beta-glucans increase fermentation in the large bowel and promote probiotic growth. This enhances the production of short-chain-fatty-acids, which are supportive of colon cell health."

**Oatstraw** — Traditionally used for arthritis, osteoporosis, sports injuries, dental decay, brittle nails and hair and for flaking or weak skin.

**Okra** — A very nutritious vegetable, being rich in B vitamins and vitamin C, as well as the minerals manganese, magnesium and potassium. It is also high in fiber and contains a plant mucin (a protein linked to a sugar — a glycoprotein — found in the secretions of mucous membranes) that soothes irritated tissue in the intestinal tract.

**Oregano Leaf** — Used traditionally for poor digestion, colic, the common cold, cough, amenorrhea (no period) and dysmenorrhea (painful periods); is an antioxidant with antifungal and antibacterial properties.

**Papaya** — Helps the digestive process.

**Parsley Leaf** — Used traditionally for cystitis, urinary spasm, prostatitis (inflammation of the prostate), edema, the common cold, amenorrhea (no period) and parturition (childbirth).

**Peppermint** — Relieves gas and spasms of the intestinal tract.

**Picrorhiza kurroa** — Used traditionally for dyspepsia, jaundice, hepatitis, cirrhosis, constipation, fever, bronchitis, asthma, allergies, inflammatory skin conditions, infection, edema, inflammatory joint disease and cancer.

**Quercetin** — A common flavonoid (plant pigment) found in many foods, including onions, grapes and green tea. It is a powerful antioxidant, which inhibits lipid peroxidation (oxidation of fatty acids), prevents GI inflammation, capillary fragility and atherosclerosis. Quercetin induces cell death in cancer cells.

**Red Clover** — Used traditionally for whooping cough, lymphadenopathy (disease affecting lymphatic system), skin disease, menopause and cancer; an expectorant and blood-purifying agent.

**Rhubarb Root** — Traditionally used in small doses for gastrointestinal irritation and for treatment of constipation and hemorrhoids.

**Slippery Elm** — Used traditionally for mucosal irritation and inflammation, wasting diseases and external wounds.

**Spearmint** — A remedy for flatulence; an antispasmodic.

**Tinaspora Cordifolia** — Used traditionally with dyspepsia, vomiting, abdominal pain, flatulence, intestinal parasites, intermittent and chronic cough, burning sensations, asthma, heart disease, hepatitis, jaundice, anemia, skin conditions, thirst, weakness, joint pain, diabetes and disorders of the genito-urinary tract.

**Triphala** — This formula from India is over 3000 years old. Triphala means "three (tri) fruits (phala)." In Ayurvedic medicine, triphala is said to cleanse the body of wastes, nourish the senses and bring about rejuvenation. Herbalists in the west commonly use it for its gentle laxative action. The three fruits contained in triphala are:

- **Emblic Myrobalan** — Used traditionally for dyspepsia, gastritis, hepatitis, pancreatitis, constipation, diarrhea, colitis, hemorrhoids, cough, asthma, hemorrhage, anemia, fever, diabetes, mental disorders, cardiovascular disease, heart disease and cancer.

- **Belleric Myrobalan** — Used traditionally for nausea, diarrhea, hemorrhage, cough, asthma, fever, prolapsed organs, bladder stones, weakness and eye diseases.

- **Chebulic Myrobalan** — Used traditionally for dyspepsia, gastroenteritis (irritation and inflammation of the digestive tract), ulcers, diarrhea, constipation, hemorrhoids, intestinal parasites, hepatosplenomegaly (enlarged liver and spleen), ascites (accumulation of fluid in the peritoneal cavity), asthma, cough, kidney stones, skin diseases, fever, joint pain, mental problems, diabetes, cardiovascular disease and cancer.

**Turmeric Root** — Used traditionally for dyspepsia, liver/gallbladder problems, liver damage, ulcers, sore throat, bronchitis, dyslipidemia (lipoprotein metabolism disorder), diabetes, skin diseases, joint pain, parasites, injuries and dysmenorrhea (painful periods); stimulates bile, protects the liver.

**Wormwood** — Used traditionally for poor digestion, colic, liver/gallbladder problems, jaundice, intestinal parasites, candidiasis, amenorrhea (no period) and leucorrhea (vaginal discharge).

**Yarrow** — Traditionally used for the common cold, fever, poor digestion, liver/gallbladder problems, poor circulation, skin diseases, chronic cystitis, amenorrhea (no period), menorrhagia (long, heavy periods), hemorrhage, wounds, bites and stings.

Yellowdock — Traditionally used for poor digestion, liver/gallbladder problems, constipation, cough, bronchitis, skin diseases and lymphatic congestion.

## AMINO ACIDS, VITAMINS & NUTRACEUTICALS

**Alpha Lipoic Acid** — A coenzyme involved in carbohydrate metabolism and in the production of adenosine triphosphate (ATP), the basic energy molecule of the cell. It has potent antioxidant activity, is both water- and fat-soluble and regenerates other antioxidants such as vitamin E, vitamin C and glutathione. Alpha lipoic acid boosts metabolism and has been shown to prevent liver damage caused by heavy metals, radiation and industrial toxins such as hexachlorobenzene. This powerful antioxidant binds with metals to help move them from the body.

**Biotin** — a B vitamin essential for normal cell growth

**Calcium D-Glucarate** — A calcium salt of D-glucarate, a form of sugar found in some vegetables and fruits, especially cruciferous vegetables, bean sprouts and apples. It assists the detoxification pathway of glucuronidation, part of the liver's Phase 2 Detoxification System. Calcium D-Glucarate helps the body excrete estrogens that can build up and promote cancerous growths. It inhibits reabsorption of toxins in bile.

**Coenzyme Q-10** — The co-factor of an enzyme — the compound necessary for the enzyme to carry out its catalytic action — a fat-soluble, vitamin-like compound involved in electron transport and energy production in the mitochondria of all cells. It is an antioxidant that is the essential component of cellular energy.

**Folic acid** — a B vitamin needed by the intestinal walls

**Fructooligosaccharides (FOS)** — Non-digestible soluble fibers that occur naturally in such foods as bananas, garlic and Jerusalem artichokes. Though half as sweet as sugar, FOS is low in calories. It is considered a "prebiotic," or food for probiotics (friendly intestinal bacteria).

**Gamma Oryzanol** — Actually a name given to a naturally-occurring group of substances derived primarily from rice bran, wheat bran and other plant foods. Gamma oryzanol has anti-inflammatory properties that make it useful in cases of gastritis, ulcers and irritable bowel syndrome. It normalizes gastric secretions and forms a protective barrier on the mucous lining of the intestines. Clinical studies show that orally administered gamma oryzanol is effective in the treatment of a broad range of gastrointestinal disorders. It has potent antioxidant activity.

**L-Glutamine** — A precursor (substance that gives rise to another substance) to glutathione, the most important antioxidant in the liver, and an essential nutrient for the cells of the small intestine (L-glutamine is their primary metabolic fuel). Glutamine deficiency has been shown to result in significant functional changes in the GI tract. Studies show that L-glutamine helps to promote healing of injured gut mucosa, making it a very important nutrient in healing a leaky gut.

**L-Glutathione** — A small molecule made up of three amino acids, which exists in almost every cell of the body. It must be generated within the cell from its precursors before it can work effectively in the body. Glutathione functions as a free radical scavenger (antioxidant) and supports Phase 2 detoxification in the liver. (See Section IV under subsection "The Liver.") It maintains immune function, enhances T-cell responsiveness and inhibits viral enzymes. Glutathione forms part of the powerful natural antioxidant glutathione peroxidase, which is found in our cells. Glutathione peroxidase plays a role in DNA synthesis and repair, metabolism of toxins and carcinogens, enhancement of the immune system and prevention of fat oxidation.

**L-Leucine** — A branched-chain essential amino acid (not made in the body, must be supplied in the diet). It ensures proper elimination of mercury once it has been bound to chelators.

**L-Methionine** — An essential amino acid that supplies elemental sulfur to the body. It plays a key role in Phase

2 reactions, assisting in the detoxification of drugs, hormones and intestinal toxins. Methionine assists in bile synthesis and has lithotiptic activity (discharges urinary and gall bladder stones).

**L-Selenomethionine** — A complex of a trace mineral (selenium) and an amino acid (methionine) that is incorporated into the enzyme glutathione peroxidase, an antioxidant and key player in Phase 2 detoxification reactions.

**L-Taurine** — A non-essential amino acid (meaning it is made in the body), often found to be deficient in the vegetarian diet. It assists in the clearance of cholesterol from the liver and stimulates bile acid synthesis. L-taurine plays a key role in Phase 2 detoxification of food preservatives and aspirin.

**Lycopene** — A fat-soluble, red-pigmented carotenoid (a family of natural pigments found in plants and animals) found in tomatoes and other fruits, including apricots, papaya, pink grapefruit, guava and watermelon. Its bioavailability is increased by application of heat (cooking) and consumption of fat. It is a potent antioxidant that may prevent cancer and deposition of fat in the arteries.

**Lutein and Zeaxanthin** — These fat-soluble, yellow-pigmented carotenoids are found in egg yolks and yellow-green vegetables and fruits. They are the only carotenoids found in the lens and retina of the eye, where they may protect against cataracts and macular degeneration. Lutein is also a major carotenoid in adipose (fat) tissue such as the breast and may help prevent cancer.

**Magnesium Hydroxide** — In large amounts, magnesium draws fluids from the bowel wall into the lumen (open space in the colon). It therefore has laxative properties. This mineral is concentrated in the heart muscle and regulates heart rhythm. It also decreases coagulation, functions as a calcium-channel blocker and relaxes smooth muscle in blood vessels.

**Methylsufonylmethane (MSM)** — An organic sulfur-containing compound and metabolite (product of metabolism) of dimethyl sulfoxide (DMSO). It is a source of sulfur for synthesis of the amino acids cysteine and methionine. Cysteine is needed in liver detoxification pathways and the synthesis of protein, and methionine is its precursor. MSM helps to restore antioxidant systems and has anti-inflammatory activity. It has been used in the treatment of interstitial cystitis (inflamed bladder wall), arthritis, gut inflammation and allergies.

**N-Acetyl-Carnitine (NAC)** — Enhances cognitive function and protects against a wide range of age-related degenerative changes in the brain and nervous system. It helps to boost energy and vitality.

**N-Acetyl Cysteine** — A precursor to glutathione production. It is a potent antioxidant. Glutathione is poorly absorbed, whereas NAC easily crosses cell membranes to form glutathione. NAC protects against damage from acetaminophen, heavy metals, pesticides and nicotine. It has anti-inflammatory properties.

**N-Acetyl-Glucosamine** — A form of glucosamine, one of the building blocks of joint tissue and other connective tissues. It is a precursor to glutamine production and may help to restore gastric and bowel integrity in inflammatory bowel disease.

**Niacin** — a B vitamin that plays a role in lowering blood cholesterol

**Pantothenic acid** — a B vitamin needed for the manufacture of hormones

**Phosphatidylcholine** — A phospholipid (a fatty substance that is a major component of cell membranes). Phosphatidylcholine prevents a decrease in membrane fluidity associated with liver disease and cancer, prevents fatty degeneration in the liver, enhances bile synthesis and has lithotriptic (dissolving or preventing stones in kidney or bladder) activity. It also delivers choline, a B vitamin that plays a key role in Phase 2 liver detoxification.

**Resveratrol** — A polyphenol with antioxidant properties that is found in greatest concentration in grape skins and red wine. It inhibits fatty deposits in blood vessels where there is inflammation, as well as cellular events associated with tumor initiation, promotion and progression. Resveratrol induces Phase 2 detoxification enzymes.

**Riboflavin** — a B vitamin that assists in the formation of new skin

**Sodium Alginate** — A sodium salt of alginic acid (an amino acid) extracted from different Laminaria species of seaweed. Commonly used as a thickener and emulsifier, sodium alginate has been shown to inhibit heavy metal uptake in the gut.

**Thiamine** — an important B vitamin; deficiency can lead to weakness, fatigue and nerve damage.

**Vitamin B6** — required for collagen (connective tissue) synthesis

**Vitamin C** — an important antioxidant that helps detoxify

*Please note: If you have followed the cleansing program in this book and have not achieved the desired results, please take the following questionnaire. If you score high please follow the candida or parasite cleansing program found in the 'Gut Solutions' book.*

# Yeast Questionnaire – Adult

## Section A – History

*Circle the number next to the questions you answer 'yes,' then add all the circled numbers and write the total in the box at the bottom.*

1. Have you taken tetracycline (Sumycin®, Panmycin®, Vibramycin®, Minocin®, etc.) or other antibiotics for acne for 1 month or more? . . . . . . . . . . . . . . . . . . . . . 50

2. Have you at any time in your life, taken other "broad spectrum" antibiotics for respiratory, urinary or other infections for 2 months or more, or for shorter periods, 4 or more times in a 1-year span? 50

3. Have you taken a broad spectrum antibiotic drug – even for 1 period? . . . . . . . . . . . . . . . . . . . . . . . . . . 6

4. Have you at any time in your life, been bothered by persistent prostatitis, vaginitis, or other problems affecting your reproductive organs? . . . . . 25

5. Have you been pregnant...
   a) 2 or more times?. . . . . . . . . . . . . . . . . . . . . . . . . . 5
   b) 1 time? . . . . . . . . . . . . . . . . . . . . . . . . . . . . . . . . . 3

6. Have you taken birth control pills for...
   a) more than 2 years? . . . . . . . . . . . . . . . . . . . . . . . . 15
   b) 6 months to 2 years? . . . . . . . . . . . . . . . . . . . . . . 8

7. Have you taken prednisone, Decadron® or other cortisone-type drugs by mouth or inhalation...
   a) for more than 2 weeks? . . . . . . . . . . . . . . . . . . . . 15
   b) for 2 weeks or less?. . . . . . . . . . . . . . . . . . . . . . . . 6

8. Does exposure to perfumes, insecticides, fabric shop odors, or other chemicals provoke...
   a) moderate to severe symptoms? . . . . . . . . . . . . . 20
   b) mild symptoms? . . . . . . . . . . . . . . . . . . . . . . . . . . 5

9. Are your symptoms worse on damp, muggy days or in moldy places? . . . . . . . . . . . . . . . . . . . . . . . . . . 20

10. If you have ever had athlete's foot, ringworm, jock itch or other chronic fungus infections of the skin or nails, have such infections been...
    a) severe or persistent?. . . . . . . . . . . . . . . . . . . . . . 20
    b) mild or moderate?. . . . . . . . . . . . . . . . . . . . . . . . 10

11. Do you crave sugar? . . . . . . . . . . . . . . . . . . . . . . . . 10

12. Do you crave breads? . . . . . . . . . . . . . . . . . . . . . . 10

13. Do you crave alcoholic beverages? . . . . . . . . . . . . 10

14. Does tobacco smoke really bother you? . . . . . . . . 10

Total Score for Section A:

_____

## Section B – Major Symptoms

*For each symptom that is present, enter the appropriate number on the adjacent line:*

- If a symptom is occasional or mild, score 3 points
- If a symptom is frequent or moderately severe, score 6 points
- If a symptom is severe and/or disabling, score 9 points

*Total the scores for this section and record them in the box at the bottom of this section.*

1. Fatigue or lethargy . . . . . . . . . . . . . . . . . . . . . . . . . ____
2. Feeling of being 'drained' . . . . . . . . . . . . . . . . . . . ____
3. Poor memory . . . . . . . . . . . . . . . . . . . . . . . . . . . . . ____
4. Feeling 'spacey' or 'unreal' . . . . . . . . . . . . . . . . . . ____
5. Inability to make decisions . . . . . . . . . . . . . . . . . . ____
6. Numbness, burning or tingling . . . . . . . . . . . . . . . ____
7. Insomnia . . . . . . . . . . . . . . . . . . . . . . . . . . . . . . . . . ____
8. Muscle aches. . . . . . . . . . . . . . . . . . . . . . . . . . . . . . ____
9. Muscle weakness or paralysis. . . . . . . . . . . . . . . . . ____
10. Pain and/or swelling in joints . . . . . . . . . . . . . . . . ____
11. Abdominal pain . . . . . . . . . . . . . . . . . . . . . . . . . . . ____
12. Constipation. . . . . . . . . . . . . . . . . . . . . . . . . . . . . . ____
13. Diarrhea . . . . . . . . . . . . . . . . . . . . . . . . . . . . . . . . . ____
14. Bloating, belching or intestinal gas. . . . . . . . . . . . ____
15. Troublesome vaginal burning, itching or discharge. . . . . . . . . . . . . . . . . . . . . . . . . ____
16. Prostatitis . . . . . . . . . . . . . . . . . . . . . . . . . . . . . . . . ____
17. Impotence . . . . . . . . . . . . . . . . . . . . . . . . . . . . . . . ____
18. Loss of sexual desire or feeling . . . . . . . . . . . . . . . ____
19. Endometriosis or infertility. . . . . . . . . . . . . . . . . . . ____
20. Cramps and/or other menstrual irregularities . . ____
21. Premenstrual tension. . . . . . . . . . . . . . . . . . . . . . . ____
22. Attacks of anxiety or crying. . . . . . . . . . . . . . . . . . ____
23. Cold hands or feet and/or chilliness. . . . . . . . . . . ____
23. Shaking or irritability when hungry. . . . . . . . . . . . ____

Total Score for Section B:

_____

## Section C – Minor Symptoms

*For each symptom that is present, enter the appropriate number on the adjacent line:*

- If a symptom is occasional or mild, score 3 points
- If a symptom is frequent or moderately severe, score 6 points
- If a symptom is severe and/or disabling, score 9 points

Total the scores for this section and record them in the box at the bottom of this section.

1. Drowsy . . . . . . . . . . . . . . . . . . . . . . . . . . . . . _____
2. Irritable or jittery . . . . . . . . . . . . . . . . . . . . . . _____
3. Lack of coordination. . . . . . . . . . . . . . . . . . . . _____
4. Inability to concentrate . . . . . . . . . . . . . . . . . _____
5. Frequent mood swings. . . . . . . . . . . . . . . . . _____
6. Headaches. . . . . . . . . . . . . . . . . . . . . . . . . . . _____
7. Dizzy/loss of balance . . . . . . . . . . . . . . . . . . . _____
8. Pressure above ear/feeling of head swelling . . _____
9. Tendency to bruise easily . . . . . . . . . . . . . . . . _____
10. Chronic rashes or itching . . . . . . . . . . . . . . . . _____
11. Psoriasis or recurrent hives . . . . . . . . . . . . . . . _____
12. Indigestion or heartburn . . . . . . . . . . . . . . . . . _____
13. Food sensitivity or intolerance . . . . . . . . . . . . . _____
14. Mucus in stools . . . . . . . . . . . . . . . . . . . . . . . . _____
15. Rectal itching. . . . . . . . . . . . . . . . . . . . . . . . . . _____
16. Dry mouth or throat . . . . . . . . . . . . . . . . . . . . . _____
17. Rash or blisters in mouth. . . . . . . . . . . . . . . . . . _____
18. Bad breath . . . . . . . . . . . . . . . . . . . . . . . . . . . . _____
19. Foot, hair or body odor not relieved by washing _____
20. Nasal congestion or post-nasal drip. . . . . . . . . _____
21. Nasal itching . . . . . . . . . . . . . . . . . . . . . . . . . . _____
22. Sore throat . . . . . . . . . . . . . . . . . . . . . . . . . . . . _____
23. Laryngitis, loss of voice . . . . . . . . . . . . . . . . . . _____
24. Cough or recurrent bronchitis . . . . . . . . . . . . . _____
25. Pain or tightness in chest . . . . . . . . . . . . . . . . . _____
26. Wheezing or shortness of breath. . . . . . . . . . . . _____
27. Urinary frequency, urgency or incontinence . . . _____
28. Burning on urination. . . . . . . . . . . . . . . . . . . . . _____
29. Spots in front of eyes or erratic vision. . . . . . . . . _____
30. Burning or tearing of eyes. . . . . . . . . . . . . . . . . _____
31. Recurrent infections or fluid in ears . . . . . . . . . . _____
32. Ear pain or deafness . . . . . . . . . . . . . . . . . . . . _____

Total Score for Section C:

GRAND TOTAL SCORE:

The total score will help you and your physician decide if your health problems are yeast-connected. A comprehensive history and physical examination are also important. In addition, laboratory studies, x-rays, and other types of tests may also be appropriate.

Scores for women will be higher, as 7 items in this questionnaire apply exclusively to women, while only 2 apply exclusively to men.

If your total score for all three sections above was less than 60 for a woman or less than 40 for a man, then you are less likely to have a problem with Candida. However, if you scored higher than this then you may wish to consider lifestyle and dietary changes, as well as a detoxification and cleansing program, all of which may help you feel healthy and more energetic.

| IF YOUR SCORE IS: | YOUR SYMPTOMS ARE: |
| --- | --- |
| 180 (women) 140 (men) | Almost certainly yeast connected |
| 120 (women) 90 (men) | Probably yeast connected |
| 60 (women) 40 (men) | Possibly yeast connected |
| below 60 (women) below 40 (men) | Probably not yeast connected |

# Yeast Questionnaire – Child

Circle appropriate point score for questions you answer "yes." Total your score and record it at the end of the questionnaire.

Point Score

1. During the two years before your child was born, were you bothered by recurrent vaginitis, menstrual irregularities, premenstrual tension, fatigue, headache, depression, digestive disorders of 'feeling bad all over?' . . . . . . . . . . . . . . . . . . . . . . . . . . . . . . . . . . . . . . . 30

2. Was your child bothered by thrush? (Score 10 if mild, score 20 if severe or persistent) . . . . . . . . . . . . . . . . . . 10/20

3. Was your child bothered by frequent diaper rashes in infancy? (Score 10 if mild, 20 if severe or persistent) . . . . . . . . . . . . . . . . . . . . . . . . . . . . . . . . . . . . . . . . . . . 10/20

4. During infancy, was your child bothered by colic and irritability lasting over 3 months? (Score 10 if mild, 20 if moderate or severe) . . . . . . . . . . . . . . . . . . . . . . . . . . . . . . . . . . . . . . . . 10/20

5. Are his/her symptoms worse on damp days or in damp or moldy places? . . . . . . . . . . . . . . . . . . . . . . . . . . 20

6. Has your child been bothered by recurrent or persistent 'athlete's foot' or chronic fungus infections of his skin or nails? . . . . . . . . . . . . . . . . . . . . . . . . . . . . . . . . . . . . . . . . . . . . . . . . . . . 30

7. Has your child been bothered by recurrent hives, eczema or other skin problems? . . . . . . . . . . . . . . . . . . . . 10

8. Has your child received:

    (a) 4 or more courses of antibiotic drugs during the past year? Or has he received continuous 'prophylactic' courses of antibiotic drugs? . . . . . . . . . . . . . . . . . . . . . . . . . . . . . . . . . . 80

    (b) 8 or more courses of 'broad-spectrum' antibiotics (such as amoxicillin, Keflex®, Septra®, Bactrim® or Ceclor®) during the past 3 years? . . . . . . . . . . . . . . . . . . . . . . . . . . . . . . . . . 50

9. Has your child experienced recurrent ear problems? . . . . . . . . . . . . . . . . . . . . . . . . . . . . . . . . . . . . . . 10

10. Has your child had tubes inserted in his ears? . . . . . . . . . . . . . . . . . . . . . . . . . . . . . . . . . . . . . . . . . . . 10

11. Has your child been labeled 'hyperactive?' (Score 10 if mild, 20 if moderate or severe) . . . . . . . . . . . . . . . . . 10/20

12. Is your child bothered by learning problems (even though his early developmental history was normal)? . . . . . . . . . . . . . . . . . . . . . . . . . . . . . . . . . . . . . . . . . . . . . . . . . . . . . . . . . . . . . . . . 10

13. Does your child have a short attention span? . . . . . . . . . . . . . . . . . . . . . . . . . . . . . . . . . . . . . . . . . . . . 10

14. Is your child persistently irritable, unhappy and hard to please? . . . . . . . . . . . . . . . . . . . . . . . . . . . . . . . 10

15. Has your child been bothered by persistent or recurrent digestive problems, including constipation, diarrhea, bloating or excessive gas? (Score 10 if mild, 20 if moderate, 30 if severe) . . . . . . 10/20/30

16. Has he/she been bothered by persistent nasal congestion, cough and/or wheezing?..................... 10

17. Is your child unusually tired or unhappy or depressed? (Score 10 if mild, 20 if servere)................10/20

18. Has your child been bothered by recurrent headaches, abdominal pain or muscle aches?
(Score 10 if mild, 20 if severe).............................................................10/20

19. Does your child crave sweets?................................................................ 10

20. Does exposure to perfume, insecticides, gas or other chemicals provoke moderate to
severe symptoms? ........................................................................... 30

21. Does tobacco smoke really bother him? ...................................................... 20

22. Do you feel that your child isn't well, yet diagnostic tests and studies haven't revealed the cause? ......... 10

TOTAL SCORE: _____

Yeasts possibly play a role in causing health problems in children with
scores of 60 or more.

Yeasts probably play a role in causing health problems in children with
scores of 100 or more.

Yeasts almost certainly play a role in causing health problems in children with
scores of 140 or more.

Reprinted from *The Yeast Connection* by William G. Crook, MD with permission.

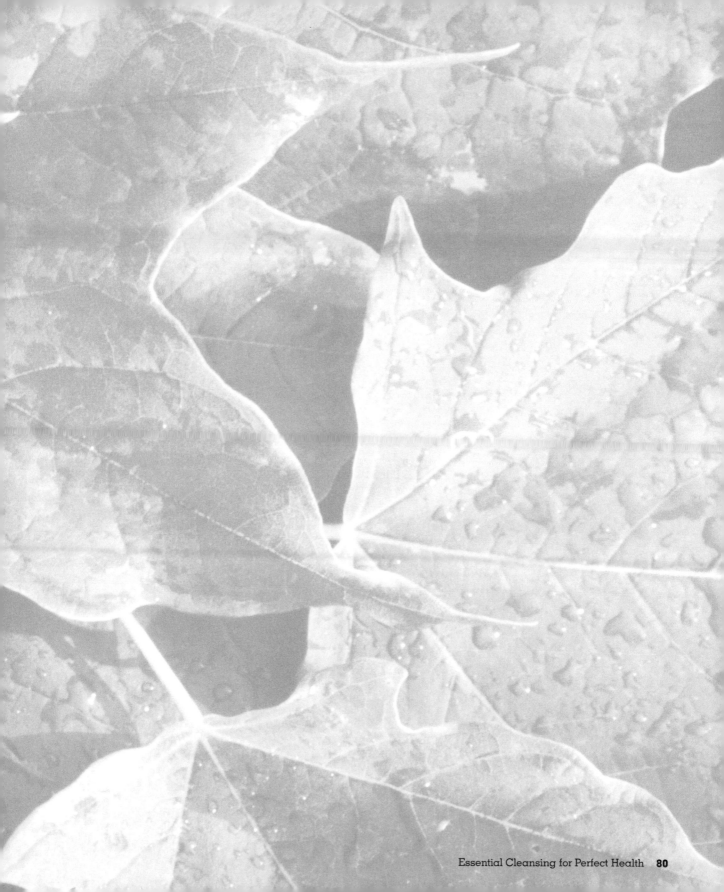